Laura Katleman-Prue's *Skinny Thinking* exposes how thought and belief can sabotage or create a healthy relationship with food and provides us with an important and empowering set of tools for transforming our relationship with how we nourish ourselves.
Georgianna Donadio, MSc, PhD
Academic Program Director
National Institute of Whole Health

FINALLY!!!! Consciousness meets food addiction. THIS BOOK IS REVOLUTIONARY! Ho, boy, am I relieved. Somebody finally wrote THE book. The book that has the possibility of truly freeing us from the bondage of food—not through another stupid diet and exercise regime, and not through another tiresome pop-psych book of feelings. What makes this book stand apart is that it goes right to the intersection of mind and mouth, where addiction kicks in, and shows you how to break that pattern with surgical precision. The strategies in this book are LIFE-CHANGING!
Lisa Holliday Lee

Skinny Thinking is an extraordinary book that guides women to a healthy weight not by providing a new fad diet, but by challenging them to permanently change their relationship with food and their bodies. Obesity is a major health problem for women and new, effective approaches are needed. Ms. Katleman-Prue teaches women how and what to eat and, more importantly, how to change the way they think about food to bring about lifelong change.
Jan L. Shifren, MD
Massachusetts General Hospital
Associate Professor of Obstetrics, Gynecology and Reproductive Biology
Harvard Medical School

My relationship with food has permanently changed! Not only am I losing weight, I know it will never come back because I look at food differently. Yea!!! I can never go back to my old ways. The steps are comprehensive and THEY WORK. I have struggled with eating and weight for years and am so delighted to have finally recovered. Your workshop and your book are the only things that have ever gotten to the root of and healed my addiction!!
Jeanne Handelman

This book provides an engaging and fun read, while offering sound advice about how thinking differently influences positive eating habits.
Gerald P. Koocher, PhD, ABPP
Dean, School of Health Sciences
Simmons College

If you truly desire to know why you overeat and want to deal with your struggles in relating to food, then this book by Laura Katleman-Prue is one you need to read.
Rev. Dr. Ed Babinsky
UCC Minister
New England Region Fitness Manager
Men's Division International

Truly unique approach to the issues of food, weight, and body image! *Skinny Thinking* is astoundingly unique, which is amazing, given the countless diet books that have been written over the past several decades. *Skinny Thinking* approaches these issues in a never-been-done-before manner by applying nondual spiritual teachings to the issues of food, weight, and body image. For me, it was the missing piece. I've spent 50+ years on the diet roller coaster and the past 15 years studying spirituality, and Laura's book, by bringing the two together, really pegged it for me—aha! moments throughout the book.
Susan Taft

I know I will read *Skinny Thinking* again and again, and I am sure I will keep getting more from it each time. The first few chapters were amazing. The idea of being free from the yo-yo is what really intrigued me. *Skinny Thinking* has gotten me to the place where I naturally make the right choices and DON'T THINK ABOUT FOOD! I have lost 12 lbs. since I started the book—I think it was five weeks ago—and I feel great. It is the wise eating and wise thinking that really clicked for me and have made life so much easier and stress free. I have been so excited about *Skinny Thinking* that I've been telling all my friends.
Susan Zipkin
Director, Radiology Research Finance
Brigham and Women's Hospital

Skinny Thinking is both inspirational and helpful. It gets to the root of self-sabotaging behaviors and then provides the necessary tools to heal them. Laura Katleman-Prue has done a great job of bringing us another way of thinking and acting in an age-old struggle.
Marcia Gorfinkle, RN, Life Coach/Stress Management Consultant

Skinny Thinking can change the life of any reader. Its novel approach represents a desperately needed breakthrough in this field.
Karen J. Puglia, MA, Psychotherapist

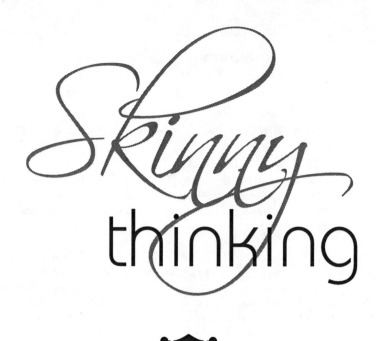

Skinny thinking

*Five Revolutionary Steps to Permanently Heal Your
Relationship with Food, Weight, and Your Body*

LAURA KATLEMAN-PRUE

New York

Skinny Thinking

Five Revolutionary Steps to Permanently Heal Your
Relationship with Food, Weight, and Your Body

Cover Design by: Rachel Lopez Rachel@r2cdesign.com

Illustrations by Laura Katleman-Prue

ISBN 978-1-60037-749-5

Library of Congress Control Number: 2010920117

Morgan James Publishing
1225 Franklin Ave., Ste. 325
Garden City, NY 11530-1693
Toll Free 800-485-4943
www.MorganJamesPublishing.com

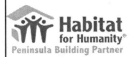
Peninsula Building Partner

In an effort to support local communities and raise awareness and funds, Morgan James Publishing donates one percent of all book sales for the life of each book to Habitat for Humanity. Get involved today. Visit **www.HelpHabitatForHumanity.org**.

To my husband Keith,
I am humbled by your unwavering love and support.
Looking into universes in your eyes is my favorite meditation.

Contents

FOREWORD

As Americans, we are all aware of the serious health crisis in this country. Obesity and our cultural obsession with food have reached epidemic proportions, not only among adults but among children and adolescents as well. Obesity-related illnesses result in hundreds of thousands of preventable deaths each year and billions of dollars in health care costs. As a cardiologist specializing in heart failure and transplantation, I see firsthand how body-weight issues impact my patients' health. Although my overweight patients are paying a terrible price for the way they are eating and living, the good news is that, for the most part, they can significantly improve their health by making even small changes in their dietary behavior.

Often, in spite of the best intentions, when people try to make changes to support a healthier way of living and eating, those changes are short-lived. The fact that more than 98% of the people who lose weight through dieting regain it within three years is clear evidence that focusing on diet, nutrition, and exercise alone is not enough to combat the problem. If we are to solve the epidemic of obesity, we must first concede that what we are doing is not working, and then embrace effective models of change. *Skinny Thinking*, a self-help book that focuses on the whole person, provides such a model.

Skinny Thinking is a remarkable compendium of tools and information that guide readers to a healthy body weight not by providing a new fad diet, but by challenging them to permanently change their relationship with food, their thinking, and their bodies. Ms. Katleman-Prue teaches people who have issues with food and body weight not only how and what to eat, but, more importantly, how to alter the way they *think* about the food they eat to bring about lifelong change.

The American health care system is failing to solve the growing pattern of obesity and other chronic conditions. The situation can only be solved by changing our health care paradigm from illness to wellness. To this end, I have begun to shift my practice toward disease prevention and self-directed wellness. I'm convinced that, ultimately, the way to achieve wellness and prevent disease is through exploring the connection between mind, body, and spirit. Among other things, I've seen the enormous impact of patients' habitual thinking patterns on their prognosis for healing once they've suffered a serious illness.

Similarly, I have no doubt that those who suffer from eating and body-weight issues engage in habitual thinking patterns that sabotage their healing efforts. This is precisely why I am excited to endorse *Skinny Thinking*. Not only is it the first book to address the role our thoughts play in health issues, it also identifies "romantic thinking" about food as the core problem. But this insightful book doesn't stop there. Because food and eating issues are complex and multifaceted, touching every aspect of life, solving them requires a whole-person approach. The *Skinny Thinking* Five Steps encompass everything from food choices, lifestyle, and eating habits, to basic emotional well-being, questioning misguided beliefs about food, and learning to connect and align with the spiritual dimension of being.

If you suffer from eating or body-weight issues and are ready to stop the cycle of yo-yo dieting, the book you now hold in your hands will provide the tools and insights you need to succeed. Just follow the simple Five Steps. My advice to every reader is if food, your body weight, or your body image is a source of worry, suffering, and ill health for you, don't delay in putting the *Skinny Thinking* Five Steps into practice.

If you devote yourself to implementing these powerful tools, you will heal your body, mind, and spirit and reap the rewards of an infinitely happier and healthier life!

Alan Gass, MD, FACC

Director of Integrative Medical Education,
National Institute of Whole Health
Director of Advanced Cardiac Failure and Transplantation,
Westchester Medical Center
Advisory Board Member, HealthCorps,
a program begun by Dr. Mehmet Oz to combat childhood obesity

ACKNOWLEDGEMENTS

Thank you, Gina Lake, for your wisdom, friendship, and encouragement, and for your incredible books! Thank you, Dr. Georgianna Donadio, for your friendship and guidance. Thank you, Dr. Bernie, for your inspiration and support. Thank you, Dr. Alan Gass, for your generous support. You epitomize the best in what health care could be. Thank you to the wonderful people at Morgan James for believing in this book: David Hancock, Rick Frishman, Lyza Poulin, and Bethany Marshall. Thank you, Eric Yaverbaum, for being such a great friend and mentor on this journey, and thank you to your extraordinary team at Ericho: Danielle Nacco, Andrea Biggs, Lauren Hovey, Mary Clare Jensen, Ilana Abel, and Danielle Pieri. Thank you to Dr. Ed Babinsky, Dr. Jan Shifren, Dr. Gerry Koocher, Karen Puglia, Marcia Gorfinkle, Jeanne Handelman, Susan Zipkin, Susan Taft, Rachel Bornstein, Lise Mousel, Darius Dahmubed, Tania Gerich, Stream Ohrstrom, Lisa Lee, Marcelle Donahue, Don Dittberner, Maudie Bremer, Melissa Linde, Barbara and Lee Cohen, Krishna Sprinkle, Helene LaMare, Meredith Miller, Amy Heller, Marcy Cohen, and Ann Marie Hartnett.

Any wisdom in these pages comes from the "deep wells" I call my teachers: Gina Lake, Theo, Stuart Schwartz, Pamela Wilson, Mooji, Michael Regan, Neelam, Adyashanti, Byron Katie, Eckhart Tolle, Nirmala, Dorothy Hunt, Ramana Maharshi, Robert Adams, Krishnamurti, Yogananda, and Nisargadatta. Last but not least, I would like to thank those whom I have not called teacher, but who have been profound way-showers nevertheless: my husband, my ex-husband, my daughter, our dog, my parents and sisters, my friends, and the greatest teacher of all—life. I bow to all of you in deep reverence and gratitude. I hope that in some small measure, this book will serve the freedom of those who read it.

INTRODUCTION

There's a way of thinking about food that's a problem, and a way of thinking about it that isn't a problem, and the problematic way corresponds to feeling out of control around food and to having a heavier body. Your *relationship with food*, which is based on how you think about it, makes all the difference. You have different relationships with your mother, your brother, your friend, your boss, and your lover, and you think about all of those people differently. In the same way, you have an easy or challenging relationship with food, depending on the way you habitually think about it.

Let's begin to explore this. How do you relate to food? As a lover, a friend, a god, an enemy, a source of nutrition? What is your image of yourself in relationship to food? What are the thoughts and self-images that mediate between you and food? When you remove all of the thoughts and images that mediate between you and food, what's left? Just a simple, pragmatic relationship with food. That is the goal of *Skinny Thinking*: to help you develop a simple, pragmatic relationship with food.

We bring so much baggage about food into the present moment that it distorts our view of food, causing us to think about and relate to it in an unhealthy way. The exercises in this book will help you unpack that baggage and see the truth about food so that you can have a simpler, wiser, and more practical relationship with it.

I know firsthand about this because food has always been my Mount Everest. If folks were ever deluded into believing that I had it all together, all they had to do was share a meal with me. If they dug a little deeper, discovered my history of dieting, and looked at the range of clothing sizes in my closet, they didn't have to be Columbo to figure out that something was off. Not only did I not have a handle on how to eat, my overeating hid a myriad of other problems, namely, repressed anger, low self-esteem, and a propensity for people pleasing.

In this book, I've included many snippets from my journey toward moderate eating and attaining a healthy weight and body image. Yet this book is not about formulating a newfangled eating or exercise plan that will deliver the perfect body to please the ego, like so many other diet books are. It is about forming a new, rational relationship with food, weight, and your body that is free from past suffering and worries. The good news is that *Skinny Thinking* is not a new fad or trend. If you put the Five Steps that you will soon learn into practice, you will keep your healthy, thinner body permanently and end the yo-yoing forever.

How to Read This Book

Please go through the book sequentially at first and begin to put the Five Steps into practice in a way that works for you. You may decide that you would rather implement the Third Step first and end with the Second Step. Or you may find that you want to do them all at the same time! The best guide for how to proceed is your own inner knowing, but if you have a health condition that requires you to eat on a certain schedule, talk to your doctor before you start implementing any of the steps. For me, a few of the steps overlapped, but they're presented here in the order that I used to become free from my compulsive eating.

Because everyone is different, we all operate on different timetables. You may be able to master the First Step right away, while your friend takes three months to complete it. And she may master the Third Step right away, while you take longer. The important thing is that you learn about the steps in order because the understanding that goes with this new relationship with food is cumulative and sequential.

Support can be helpful on this journey. Get hooked up with a buddy through the Facebook fan group SKINNY THINKING! By Laura Katleman-Prue. Then, log on to the *Skinny Thinking* website (www.SkinnyThinking.com) to sign up for the e-newsletter. Check out the website calendar for the *Skinny Thinking* Workshop, conference call, and podcast schedules.

The *Skinny Thinking* Approach

This approach is about learning to align with your true nature rather than with the false self, or ego. When you are in touch with what I call *the true self* or *the Wise Witness*, you are in touch with a mature, wise part of you at the core of your being. When you are aligned with that, rather than with the ego, or negative thoughts that constantly chatter in your head, you feel happy and at peace. The ego experiences separation from other people and creates the fear at the root of your suffering, including your eating-related suffering. When you are identified with the ego instead of the Wise Witness, you innocently make choices that are contrary to your physical, psychological, and spiritual well-being.

By using the Five Steps, you will see that when you're identified with the ego, you relate to food from your conditioning, and this causes you to look for things from food that it cannot provide. From this place, you may overeat or eat the wrong foods because your uninvestigated thoughts are mediating between food and you. The ego tempts you with a thin sliver of truth, the pleasurable aspect of eating, and filters out everything else. Then, based on this slant, it creates desires and drives that interfere with a simple and natural relationship with food. Those desires and drives impel you to reach for food whether you're hungry or not, and before you know it, the pounds are piling on.

But when you're able to drop out of the ego and move into alignment with the Wise Witness, those thoughts disappear, and you're able to see a pure, practical way of eating that's based on food's true function. This natural way of relating to food includes the entire picture—"the whole truth about food."

You can become free from ego-based distortions and overblown desires by not listening to the thoughts that create them and by seeing them for what they are, conditioning that keeps us imprisoned in egoic consciousness and suffering.

Although this book is about healing eating and body-image issues, it has another potential benefit—helping you experience who you really are beyond the ego. As much as your troubled relationship with food may have been the bane of your existence, your suffering has motivated you to pick up this book and has brought you to an exciting watershed in your evolution: realizing that your ego has been lying to you for years. Your willingness to see the truth makes permanent healing a real possibility and turns a wonderfully hopeful new page in the story of your journey.

If it does its job, *Skinny Thinking* will act like smelling salts, waking you up from your food nightmare. My promise to you is that if you keep an open mind and are willing to put the Five Steps into practice, this will be the last book you will ever have to read on this subject. Weight and food worries will become relics of the past. Once and for all, you will finally make peace with the eating and body-image issues that have plagued you, and experience the freedom that is your birthright.

CHAPTER 1

Freedom Is Possible

• ◆ •

Yes, it is possible to be free from your obsession with food and body weight! It is possible to live without worrying about what you will eat next and whether it will make you fat, or if you'll have the willpower to eat in a way that keeps you from busting out of your jeans. It is possible to free yourself from troubles with food that cause a myriad of health problems, including weight gain. It is possible to live without measuring your self-worth by the vicissitudes of the bathroom scale. It is possible to leave this seemingly insurmountable source of suffering behind.

Not only is this possible—you're already halfway there! By reading this book, you've taken the single most important step, without which no healing is possible: You've decided that you don't want to suffer anymore. In effect, you've said, "Enough already!" You're ready to find a way out.

Your suffering has led you to want freedom more than you want your old habits. You're ready to end your romantic relationship with food, to stop seeing it primarily as a source of pleasure and entertainment rather than as nice-tasting nutrition, and to finally be free. And this is indeed a freedom book, not just the usual diet book that's focused solely on losing weight. It will help you create new habits, which will allow you to lose weight and keep it off this time. Although the information in this book may not necessarily be what you want to hear, if you really want to be free, and not just continue to yo-yo, you have to change your relationship to food fundamentally and permanently. If you do that, you'll be free from torment and have the healthy body that you want.

The purpose of this book is to help you see *the whole truth about food* and what's been going on in your relationship with it. No matter how long you've been struggling with food, you don't have to take this issue to your grave. You can free yourself of it for good. All you have to do is follow the Five Steps.

In the upcoming pages, you'll see how your thinking has led to an overblown relationship with food and that this relationship is the root of your weight issues. You will discover that romanticizing food leads to being overweight, and that looking in the mirror from your ego's perspective reinforces body identification and causes suffering. Thankfully, there is another way: moving out of ego-based thinking and into the Wise Witness. This way of being sets you free and leaves worries about weight in the distant past.

Freedom Exercise

This exercise will help you imagine the life you would have if you took back your power over food:

> *Close your eyes and get in touch with the impact of food and weight issues in your life. What have they cost you physically, mentally, emotionally, and spiritually? How have they impacted your self-esteem and your relationships? Have they kept you from following your heart and going after what you've wanted?*
>
> *Now imagine how your life would be if you felt free and relaxed around food. Imagine that it no longer absorbs your mental energy. You no longer feel powerless or afraid, but aligned, balanced,*

centered, and confident. How would you live? How would you treat yourself and others? Imagine all of the energy that you used to devote to worrying and thinking about food flowing into creative and fulfilling endeavors in your life. How does your body feel? Notice any emotions or sensations that arise.

Use this exercise as often as you can, even once a day, to support the permanent change you're making in your relationship to food.

This exercise shows you the cost of your romantic relationship with food and what would be possible if thoughts about food no longer dominated your life. I promise you, there is life after your love affair with food! A rich life replete with the benefits that come from living in a healthy body and in alignment with a fulfilling life purpose, a life in which food thoughts no longer take center stage. From now on, when a pesky food thought is on the scene and you're tempted to follow it, ask yourself, "Is it worth it? Is it worth giving up my freedom to follow this thought? What is my freedom really worth?"

Why Are Food and Weight Issues So Tough?

Why are food, weight, and body-image issues so intransigent? The quick-and-dirty answer is: We're programmed to listen to and believe our thoughts. In the case of food and weight, our egoic mind pits two stubborn, mutually exclusive desires against each other: the desire to experience taste pleasure from food and the desire to look good. No wonder we're in a pickle! On the one hand, our bodies need food to survive and we're programmed to adore food. On the other hand, we're bombarded with media images of young, thin, attractive people and brainwashed into thinking that we should look that way, too.

We're like pendulums swinging from one end of the desire-fulfillment scale to the other. First, we indulge our desire to eat for pleasure, which causes us to gain weight. Then, we feel miserable because we've failed to satisfy our desire for thinness. Next, we diet, lose weight, and feel deprived of the foods we love. Our deprivation causes us to desire pleasure foods (foods with little or no nutrition that are ultimately not fulfilling), and eventually, we give in, overeat, and gain weight again. Our weight gain brings us full circle, causing the desire to be thin to kick in again, and on and on it goes.

Living between these two competing desires is quite a conundrum—for everyone but the ego. As long as we have a problem, the ego has a job. It's in the problem-creation-and-solution business. For those of us who have food and weight issues, it's a full-time job. Once we're hooked, the ego can just kick back and sip a piña colada, having achieved its goal of ensnaring us in constant problems in order to keep itself employed.

The good news is that the food and weight issues that have been the bane of your existence are also your custom-designed ticket to freedom. The question is: Will you use it? Are you ready to be done with this issue once and for all? Are you willing to try something new? Are you ready to have a healthy relationship with food and your body? If your answer is yes, the principles presented here can free you. All you have to do is let go of any preconceptions and memories of past failures, and open your heart and mind to receiving new information through both these pages and your own intuition.

Is This Another Diet?

Whenever I utter the word "diet," people fidget in their seats, their faces harden, and they say, "Oh no—not me. I'm not going there." But before your shutters slam shut, please let me explain.

Skinny Thinking is not a diet; it's about creating a new relationship to food that automatically results in greater health and a healthier weight. Diets are temporary. People are willing to stick to them for a while in order to lose weight, but then they stop and go back to their old habits.

The goal of *Skinny Thinking* is to change your fundamental relationship to food by changing how you habitually think about it. If you don't do that, you might as well hang it up right now. No diet, no matter how vigilant you are, is going to work long term without that component.

Relax. I'm not asking you to go on yet another diet. Instead, I'm encouraging you to:

1. Permanently change your diet and
2. Change your relationship to food.

Let's take these one at a time. Changing your diet means changing what you're eating habitually so that most of your calories come from healthy, nutritious, whole foods, and eating those foods in reasonable portions.

The second component is changing your relationship to food. Bad eating habits in part stem from the way you've been thinking about food. Hence, the diet I advocate is a "thought diet," questioning and debunking the fantasies that have been mediating between you and food.

When it comes right down to it, skinny thinking is a truth-telling exercise to bust through your illusions and beliefs about food. Ultimately, you must begin to let go of deluded, misguided beliefs and your romanticized relationship with food in order to stop suffering and yo-yoing. In my experience, the best tool to achieve this is inquiry.

To recap, neither component can work without the other. Merely changing the foods you eat and your portion sizes isn't enough. Neither is changing your relationship to food if you're still getting the bulk of your calories from junk and eating unreasonably large portions. A bird needs both of its wings to fly, and healing your food issues requires both components to be complete and lasting—a shift in your diet and a change in your relationship with food.

The truth can't be changed, because the truth is always the truth. You can't continue to eat the way you've been eating and have the healthy body you want. It's simple and unambiguous. Yet many of us have been in denial, pretending that it isn't so. We want to look good, feel good, and keep eating all the junk we want. C'est impossible!

It's natural to look for a way to somehow have your cake and eat it, too, to somehow maintain your bad habits and still enjoy a healthy, slim body. It seems like other people can do it, right? Why not you? But do you really know what other people are doing to maintain thin bodies while they scarf down massive slabs of chocolate fudge cake?

Very few people can eat whatever they want and stay thin. Even if they manage to stay thin, what are the health consequences of eating all that junk? Once again, the truth is still the truth: You have to change your old habits if you want to heal this issue. Only then will you start to reap the rewards.

If you trade your old eating and thinking habits for healthy ones, over time you will naturally settle into a healthy weight. Rather than focusing on a goal weight, as you might have done when you were dieting, focus on not going back to your old habits.

You might as well just bite the bullet. Look yourself squarely in the eyes and tell yourself the truth: "_____, you can never go back to your old habits and stay thin." This is the truth that most people don't want to face.

To be really free, you have to transform your relationship to food forever. You have to be willing to change the way you eat and think about food and never go back. That's the simple, kind truth of it. Now go forth and heal! You can do this!

My Story

From the age of 16, when I went on my first real diet, until I was 49, I succumbed to the cultural imperative to "be the best I could be" by dieting, and my life traced the self-worth-negating arc of the overeating-dieting pendulum. Like the rising and setting sun, my eating cycles were so predictable, you could set a clock by them. This inevitable oscillation was a safe haven that allowed me to postpone my life until I had the right body size to create a successful life.

Dieting led to overeating, and overeating led to yet another diet. This is the cycle of desperation, hope, elation, deprivation, indulgence, and self-flagellation you sign on for when you listen to the ego's perspective about food and life. When you decide for the umpteenth time to go on another diet without permanently changing your relationship with food, you delude yourself into believing, despite ample evidence to the contrary, that this will be the one that works.

One of the reasons it was so hard to maintain my weight, in spite of all my dieting, was that the intensity of my love affair with chocolate equaled my desire to have a thin body. In my early 20s, this love had its business advantages. Because I couldn't think of anything I loved more than chocolate, it was easy to follow the advice laid out in entrepreneurship books: Sell a product you're excited about. It was a no-brainer. Brownies, the richest, chocolatiest dessert I could think of, would be my product— and voila! The Boston Brownie Company was born.

For a certified chocoholic, my new business was heaven, a dream come true. Like an addict suddenly finding herself with an unending supply of her drug of choice, my cup runneth over. I filled my days sampling gourmet chocolates, swirling them into rich batters, and baking them to sinful, gooey perfection, all in the noble service of offering the public the most perfect brownies. Who says that being an adult is no fun?

Having spent my childhood using food as a source of comfort and pleasure, it was natural for me to parlay this food focus into a business. Unknowingly, I'd developed an addictive relationship with sugar and chocolate, and now my new business gave me an excuse to keep my fridge stocked with a delicious combination of both—brownies.

To other people, starting a business like this was not only adaptive, it was laudable. I was a 20th-century woman, exemplifying the pioneering spirit that made our country great. Certainly, that spin sounded a heck of a lot better than "I am an addict getting my daily fix!"

Eating Is a Messy Business

After a less than stellar performance at my college dance recital, my best friend, Lisa, tried to reassure me that I had done fine. But I knew better. Lisa was in best-friend mode, doing what friends are supposed to do—help their buddies feel better by sugarcoating the truth. Whether I'd blown it or not, what mattered was that I was upset with my performance. Convinced that I'd humiliated myself, the experience reinforced my core belief that I couldn't do anything right.

Lisa, partner in crime and eating buddy extraordinaire, and I decided that there was only one thing to do: help me escape my perceived public humiliation by eating up one side of the town and down the other. Like a lover planning a secret tryst, we excitedly choreographed our plan for procuring the forbidden object of our lust—pleasure food. Starting at the local coffee shop, we crammed down grilled cheese sandwiches (of all things!) at warp speed. After the sandwiches, I felt full, but stopping was not an option. No, by gosh, we were on a mission—a mission of avoidance, and central to that mission was eating ourselves senseless. That evening, we would stuff ourselves with large quantities of the naughty foods we denied ourselves the rest of the time.

For a few short hours, I believed that bingeing would help me avoid feeling like a failure. I hoped that if I ate massive quantities of food, I would numb or avoid the powerful, messy emotions that left me feeling helpless, hopeless, and most of all, out of control.

After the grilled cheese sandwiches, we sped off to our signature bingeing destination: Foster's, an all-night donut shop. Salivating as we peered through the window, our eyes met a confectionary vision of perfectly shaped cruller soldiers, nobly sacrificing themselves into an enormous vat of boiling oil. The flimsy sticks emerged seconds later, metamorphosed by the baptism, inflated to twice their original size. Then, for the pièce de résistance, a pudgy, apron-clad man cavalierly scooped them up and deposited them onto sugar-encrusted racks.

Although we were charmed by the array of beguiling donuts and crullers before us, Lisa and I remained loyal to our favorite treat: apple fritters. They weren't pretty. In fact, if you didn't know any better, you might take fritters for defective outcasts, the unfortunate result of a donut mishap. These misshapen, brown blobs looked more like weapons than donuts—crusty points jutting out in all directions. Only the sheen of their sugar glazing gave them away as purposefully designed treats.

Fritters were not for the faint of heart—only a truly intrepid binger dared indulge in these enigmas. When pierced, their strange outer crust revealed a soft, breadlike interior delicately veined with syrup-drenched chunks of apple. Somewhere, a donut genius had conceived the perfect taste and textural complement to a fritter's crusty outer shell. Suffice it to say that no Foster's run was complete without a box of fritters, and as a matter of principle, sort of a binger's code of ethics, fritters never made it home.

Pretending to be throwing a party, Lisa also ordered boxes of warm, gooey donuts, casually tossing in comments like "Bobby loves this one. Tony wants that one. Let's get three of those…" in order to divert attention from the embarrassing truth—that our party was actually a party of two.

Visits to Foster's were never casual. There was a frenzied hyperactivity to our trips there, and this night was no different. Laden with donut boxes, we headed off to buy pizza and ice cream. Two hours after we began our eating rampage, we triumphantly sped back to the dorm.

At school, we went into stealth mode, transferring our booty from the car to Lisa's room undetected. After lining up our feast picnic-style on the floor, we ate ourselves into oblivion. Rhythmically stuffing ourselves with a practiced precision, we entered a food-numbed trance, anesthetizing ourselves from painful thoughts and feelings, pretending that we could escape life's disappointments—and there was some truth to this because for some part of those few hours, we did escape. We did control our lives by exchanging emotional pain for physical pain, at least for the moment, until we had to face the triple whammy: the painful emotions that precipitated the binge, the guilt over the loss of willpower evidenced by the binge, and our imminent weight gain.

Hours later, our binge wound down, and the food we'd longed for and fantasized about was now repulsive. Sleep arrived, mercifully sparing us any further protests from our swollen bellies. There we lay until daylight—stuffed and exhausted, trapped in a maze of boxes that revealed an array of half-eaten, waxy donuts and congealed pizza slices.

Having a Party with Food

A binge party like mine doesn't happen out of the blue. I had a history, beliefs, and perceived needs that led to my out-of-whack relationship with food. As a child, I had learned to numb out with food. Because this was my pattern, when I felt uncomfortable emotions on the night of my college dance recital, it wasn't a surprise that I turned to food to escape from them. Because my drug of choice had always been food, at the first sign of an unwanted emotion, I dove headfirst into sweet, fatty, starchy, or salty food, swallowing the food so fast that I barely chewed, much less tasted it. Distracted by the angry, fearful, or worrisome thoughts that precipitated my frenzied eating, I entered a trance, making it easy to miss the actual experience of eating. One after another, the negative thoughts wove an evermore compelling and upsetting story, intensifying the feelings and leading to more unconscious, frantic, compulsive eating.

Caught in the talons of stressful thoughts, eating was the only way I knew to take care of myself. The thoughts seemed so logical and true that it didn't occur to me that I could ignore them. Instead, I would throw myself a binge party to anesthetize the pain of the upsetting feelings created by my negative thoughts.

There are parties with food, and there are PARTIES! We can have a small party or an over-the-top party. The more stressed out and out of balance we are, the more likely we'll have a party that is out of balance and, ultimately, unsatisfying. We can have a party with food in moderation, and there's no harm done, but *binge parties are not parties at all* in the end.

Bingeing begins with a desperate, empty feeling that leads to an uncontrollable desire to eat pleasure food. Entering a hypnoticlike state, we're unable to stop gorging even after we've become uncomfortable or sick. Bingeing has a self-destructive, unconscious component that's connected to repressed emotions and can represent an unconscious motivation to hurt the body.

If you're bingeing, I recommend working with a skilled, empathic psychotherapist. The information in this book can be a helpful adjunct to psychotherapy. Psychotherapy teaches you to accept and positively express your feelings, needs, desires, and drives. Learning not to repress anger or drives, including egoic drives, is basic emotional hygiene—the step before going beyond the mind and the emotions.

You don't have to be bingeing, though, to benefit from the Five Steps. If, like many people, you find yourself eating when you're not hungry, it's likely that you're using food to get happy, and you can learn to change that habit. Eating when you're not hungry creates a cycle of suffering: You eat to get happy, feel bad for indulging, and then eat more to escape your emotional discomfort. I'm sure you'll agree—this isn't the most constructive strategy.

Why Me?

Why was I given eating and body-image issues that have caused me untold suffering? If the answer is that these issues lead to growth, it's fair to ask, "Who set up this sadistic system where suffering leads to growth?"

At first, it can feel like a cruel joke of the Creator. Does He or She delight in our pain as we get on and off the dieting merry-go-round? How could suffering with eating and body-image issues be a good thing? The truth is that eventually, if we're lucky, this suffering becomes so unbearable that we're no longer willing to experience it. We come to a crossroads and decide that we're not willing to live this way anymore. We set off in search of books like this one to help us recognize the fallacy of painful beliefs that tell us food is the be all and end all and that our bodies should look better than they do.

Like touching a hot stove over and over again and deluding ourselves into believing we won't get burned this time, we continue to turn to food for things it can't give us and berate ourselves for how our bodies look. Yet body and eating issues can actually help us see our way to a happier life once we realize that the way we've been thinking and living doesn't serve us. The stressful issues that dog us year after year are most instrumental in catalyzing our growth. Even though they hurt like heck, they're ultimately our ticket to freedom from suffering.

The Ego and the True Self in the Battle of the Bulge

The epic conflict enacted under the guise of the battle of the bulge is the struggle between the ego, that negative chatterbox in our heads, and the true self. It's the suffering caused by this battle that moves us to break free from our unconscious patterns and conditioning and instead live from the true self. In this state, we are free to experience the peace and joy available in each moment. This is the battle: resistance versus acceptance; the ego versus the true self; self-delusion versus truth; the ego's small sliver of truth about food and the body versus the whole picture.

The Villain

The villain in our story, the ego, has three faces: the Critic, the Child, and the Dreamer. In our struggles with body image, the ego in the form of the relentless Critic is the judgmental voice inside our head berating the way our body looks, telling us, "You're too fat"; "Your chest is too small"; "Your thighs are too big"; "You need to look like the images you see in the media—young, thin, and beautiful"; and "You'll never attract the kind of relationship you want unless you get into better shape."

When it comes to food, the pleasure-seeking Child causes us to gain weight by telling us things like: "You've been working so hard, you deserve a slice…or two…or three of cheesecake"; "You should live a little. Give yourself a treat"; "Eating a bit more won't hurt"; "You've had a lousy day, so why not make yourself feel better with a little pleasure food?"; and "Indulge now and worry about tomorrow tomorrow."

The ego is a lot of things, but it's no fool. To stay employed, it invented the never-ending "build-a-better me" project. Here's how it works: The Child creates our eating problem by tempting us to use pleasure food as a treat, cajoling us to eat a few more bites even when our stomachs are bursting. Then, the Critic has the unmitigated gall to shame and castigate us over the weight gain the Child caused!

The coup de grace comes as we're sobbing into our Häagen Dazs carton, looking to escape the misery of a belly that overflows our jeans. That's when the ego in the form of the Dreamer rides in on a white steed, offering salvation—a new diet that will rid us of our excess weight and let us become the sexy vixens we've always known we could be. It declares that we still have a chance to win the love and attention of the perfect prince or princess and live a happy life. Just when our storybook ending is within reach, the Child appears again, enticing us with momentary taste pleasure. When we fall off the wagon due to the Child's incessant luring, the Critic will be there to chastise us, and when we feel sufficiently beaten down, the Dreamer offers salvation— and we're off and running again.

As you can see, the ego really knows how to keep us busy and distracted. We can become so caught up in trying to hurdle its eating and weight-loss obstacles that we don't realize that it's causing our suffering. Once we stop listening to the ego and doing its bidding, we immediately experience the pure joy of just being. This is exactly what the ego wants to keep from us because once we discover we don't need it to be happy, the ego's out of a job. But we can take our power back and choose instead to rest in the peace and contentment that's available in every moment in the natural state of the true self. The more we do this, the more time we spend in the true self, the easier it is to heal our eating issues and lose weight.

The Hero

Now that we've seen the villain in our story, it's time to get to know our hero, the true self, or the Wise Witness. The Wise Witness *is* our true self, the one who naturally knows what to eat to keep us healthy. It's who we are when we're not listening to and believing in the ego. It's that inner place of calm and serenity that we've all visited in moments when the mind is quiet. Think back to a time when you've felt completely at peace. That delicious feeling is the true self. Even though we may not be aware of this consciously, each of us taps into it every day!

We can see the true self clearly in the innocence and openness in babies and animals. They're the true self embodied. I'm not suggesting returning to the pre-egoic state but, rather, that if we want to experience life from a delightful place of openness, wonder, and curiosity, we have to relearn how to connect with the true self, shedding what no longer serves us so that our natural state of radiant happiness shines through.

Connecting with the Wise Witness means entering the thought-free state beyond identification with our minds and bodies. Although meditation is the most common way to move out of the mind, we can do this anywhere, anytime, as long as we're not caught up in thoughts or feelings. We can notice the clock on the wall, a leaf floating in the breeze, or our hand as we turn the page.

When you are in the ego-based state of consciousness, thoughts and feelings come between you and direct experience. For example, you're in the true self, in a moment of awe, when you see a beautiful sunset—and when thought comes in, saying, "Oh, what a beautiful sunset," you're back in the ego.

Information we receive from the senses, before thought comes in, takes us to the true self. If we are to break the habit of paying attention to and following our thinking, which is responsible for our food issues, it helps to cultivate a new habit of diving into the space between our thoughts. To do that, try to spend at least 10 to 15 minutes every day sitting quietly, either in silence or while listening to restful music.

Conditioning

Our conditioning is made up of painful beliefs we innocently formed in childhood to protect ourselves. Not only do these beliefs no longer serve us, they keep us from our natural happiness. Given this, there are two reasons we might overeat even a healthy food:

1. To nurture ourselves.
2. To "stuff our feelings"—to use food to medicate ourselves and avoid having to experience our feelings.

In both cases, we overeat because our conditioning has been triggered, either by an event or by our negative thinking. But with this triggering comes an opportunity to become free from it once and for all. The First Step, Wise Thinking, which you will learn about in the next chapter, shows you how to heal conditioning by questioning your old beliefs and stepping back into awareness.

There are two ways to approach eating: from the Child's point of view (our conditioning, which is part of the ego) or from the true self's point of view. Whenever we're eating to fill a psychological need rather than a physical need, we're identifying with our conditioning. The true self, on the other hand, encourages actions that support the optimal functioning of the body, so it's unlikely that the true self will move us to overeat when we've had enough.

The voice of the ego can be loud and harsh or seductive and cajoling. Following it moves us into its painful, damned-if-you-do, damned-if-you-don't world. The ego seduces us into eating too much of the wrong foods, and then berates us afterwards. Anything to control us! Luckily, just because it is trying to tempt us doesn't mean we have to pay attention to it. We are in control of our attention, and if we don't like what's playing on ego radio, we can simply turn it off and drop into the true self. Here are some examples of how the Child tries to get us to eat when the body isn't hungry:

❀ I love this taste. I want more of it.

✦ I'll be hungry later if I stop now.

✦ That tastes really good. Just a bite or two more won't hurt.

✦ This is healthy, so I can eat more of it. So what if I'm not really hungry anymore?

✦ I've been good; I deserve that second dessert.

✦ I'm bored. What can I eat now?

✦ I should be hungry now. It's dinnertime, so I might as well eat something.

When we have overindulged, the Critic berates us with harsh judgments such as:

✦ You know you shouldn't have eaten that; now you'll gain weight.

✦ You are such a glutton.

✦ It wasn't enough to eat some of that; you had to go and eat the whole thing!

✦ You're insatiable.

✦ Eating like that is a sin. Repent or God will send you to hell.

✦ You'll never get the body you want this way, and then you'll die fat, unhappy, and alone.

When you notice that you're eating to fill a psychological need, simply being aware of it can shift you back into the true self. _When you're able to notice your conditioning, you stop identifying with the ego and start identifying with the true self._ It's that simple. Noticing it is all it takes.

Becoming aware of your conditioning opens up the possibility of another choice. Rather than following the well-worn path of emotional eating, you can choose _not_ to do that. You can ask yourself, "Is this really what I want to be doing right now? Will it satisfy me forever?" This moves you out of identification with your conditioning and into the true self, your own inner wisdom.

We're also in the ego whenever we eat without any conscious connection to food or the body. We eat unconsciously when we're either caught up in thought or in the midst of an emotional upset. Neither is a good time to eat because we can't pay attention to how full we're getting. Before we know it, the body is stuffed, and we haven't fully experienced or enjoyed the experience of eating.

The ego is the voice of the extreme. On one hand, it advocates excess and indulgence and on the other, rigid restriction or deprivation. Whenever eating results in suffering, we know we're in the ego.

In contrast, the true self advocates balance, health, and temperance. It's quiet and doesn't fight for our attention, but nudges us and speaks to us through our intuition. For example, when we're grocery shopping, we may feel moved to buy something healthy that wasn't on our shopping list. This subtle nudging is from the true self, moving us in a direction that serves the body's well-being.

Bringing Awareness to Eating and How You Think about Food

When it comes to seeing through the negative beliefs that cause you to bolt toward the fridge, start by bringing more awareness to your eating. Are you aligned with the ego or the true self when you pick up a fork? Are you engrossed in thought or are you present, experiencing directly whatever is happening now?

To align with the true self, continually bring your attention back to *awareness* by asking yourself, "What's happening in this moment?" It should come as no surprise that awareness is key in healing our dysfunctional relationship with food. Whenever we are aware, rather than listening and paying attention to thoughts, we're aligned with the true self, and the ego has no power over us.

For years, you may have been innocently overeating because that's how you learned to comfort and take care of yourself when you were feeling bad. Dating back to childhood, overeating to get happy and stuff uncomfortable feelings may have been how you loved yourself.

Now you see that this way of caring for yourself doesn't serve you and creates suffering rather than happiness and comfort.

An important part of this process is discovering what food means to you. What is the emotional connection you've created with food? Are you actually present when you're eating? It's easy to become hypnotized by the rhythmic motion of your fork or get lost in thoughts or emotions, paying little or no attention to how much you're putting in your tank. No wonder it's easy to gain weight! Eating without being present is like pumping gas blindfolded from a tank with no automatic shut-off. Neither has a good outcome. One brings a messy gas spillover, the other, a belly spillover.

Awareness Tips

Ironically, those of us who love food and see it as central to our happiness are not very aware when we're eating. We find ourselves eating quickly or while doing something else, such as driving, talking on the phone, watching television, or reading, so the experience of eating isn't as satisfying as it could be.

Begin to bring awareness to the whole process of eating by getting curious about it. When and why do you decide to eat something? What are your eating triggers? How are you feeling while you're eating? Are you engaged in the experience of eating, or is your mind somewhere else, engaged in problem solving or ruminating over a frustrating experience? Follow these next steps to help you begin to bring more awareness to your eating:

1. **Set the intention.** Set the intention to bring awareness to your eating and your thoughts about food. Once you have set an intention to understand more about your eating, be prepared for insights to arise.

2. **Notice eating triggers.** How does eating happen for you? How do you decide when and what to eat? Start to notice your eating

triggers. What are you thinking, feeling, or believing when the idea of eating something pops in? What are the emotions and thoughts that send you racing toward the fridge? When you're bored, is your first impulse to get some food?

3. **Be aware of portion size.** Become aware of how much food you're putting on your plate. Is it a reasonable amount? Many of us are used to eating portions that are much larger than we need.

4. **Be aware of other activities while eating.** What are you doing when you're eating? Are you driving, surfing the Internet, watching television, or having a heated discussion?

5. **Notice your thoughts.** What are you thinking about? Are you anxious about paying your bills? Are you replaying an uncomfortable conversation from earlier in the day?

6. **Be aware of your feelings.** What are you feeling? Are you stressed, anxious, angry, or fearful? Does the life you're living suit you? Are you doing what you love to do? If your overall choices aren't right for you, you're going to feel depressed, and that depression will fuel your food issues.

7. **Take some notes.** Record any insights or images that come to mind.

I suspect that you're reading this book because you're looking for change on a deeper level, beyond just going on a diet—you were moved by the evolutionary impulse for freedom. When we shine the light of our awareness on how we eat and think, it opens the door to a permanent change that transforms our life on every level. We become happier, freer, and more fulfilled.

In the upcoming chapters, you will learn the Five Steps that helped me free myself from my eating and body-image issues. They're not a quick fix, but they do work if you give them a chance. If you approach them with an open mind and put them into practice, your time and effort will be rewarded many times over.

CHAPTER 2
The First Step: Wise Thinking

• ◆ •

Congratulations! You are about to take the first step on your exciting journey toward freedom and healing. Imagine how you'll feel when you arrive. Worries about food and your weight will be relics of your past. What a relief! If you put the Five Steps into practice, I promise you that that feeling of freedom will be your everyday experience.

The First Step, Wise Thinking, is my all-time favorite because it was the last nail in my food-and-weight-issues coffin. It was the important understanding that I had been missing. If you truly want to heal your food and weight issues, Wise Thinking is the opportunity you've been waiting for. Skip it and you'll keep yo-yoing and miss the chance to heal permanently.

To fully embrace Wise Thinking means creating an entirely new, healthy relationship with food. Get ready to learn how to think *differently* about food and, hopefully, think very little about it, if at all, when it's not time to eat. In this chapter, you'll learn helpful strategies to stop wearing a path to the fridge, such as recognizing when the Child is on the scene and learning to ignore her, seeing the whole picture of food, and implementing kung fu for cravings and emotional eating. Fasten your seatbelt because you're about to blast through the barriers that have held these issues in place!

How Do You Think about Food?

How do you think about food? How often do you think about it? When do you think about it? Do you think more about food when you're tired, bored, sad, lonely, or stressed out? What is your personal relationship with food? What are your mental representations of it? What does food mean to you beyond nutrition and fuel? It's important to get very clear about this because if you're thinking about food as anything other than nice-tasting fuel, you need to change your thinking in order to heal your relationship with it.

Take a moment to write down the answers to these questions in a journal, and then revisit your answers over the next few days and weeks. Become aware of your food thoughts and the situations that trigger them. Notice what's happening when the idea of eating arises and you're not physically hungry, and then record your discoveries in your journal.

Just about now you may be thinking, "What's the big deal about food thoughts? They're just thoughts. You can't see them or touch them. Why do they matter so much?" The big deal is that if you're still listening to them and following them rather than ignoring them, they are the core of your eating struggles and suffering.

When I first began my own healing journey, I realized that I thought about food constantly. As soon as I learned how to ignore those thoughts, they arose less and less often, and food and being overweight ceased to be issues for me.

If you're eating too much, eating the wrong foods, or both, you're thinking a lot about food. If you want your actions to change, you have to change the root cause of those actions—the way you think about food.

Thoughts lead to feelings and feelings lead to actions. The way you think about food creates certain feelings and those feelings lead to eating. You can force off weight by going on a diet, but just like when you pull off the top of a weed, the problem will come right back if you don't take care of the root.

To permanently heal your eating issues and stop struggling with your weight, you have to change your relationship with food by changing the way you think about it.

How Does Skinny Thinking Work?

Can you restrict your thoughts about food the same way you restrict your calories on a diet? To stop thinking about food may seem about as possible as refraining from eating altogether. When food has been your primary source of pleasure and nurturance, to stop thinking about it seems inconceivable. Therein lies the rub. We *assume* that it's not possible, so we don't even try.

Luckily, a thought about food is just a thought, like any other. In and of themselves, thoughts have no power. I repeat, *thoughts have no power*—none, nada, zilch! The ego wants you to believe that you can't ignore a food thought and that you have to follow it, that once a food thought is on the scene, you have to find and consume pleasure food right away. But that is just the Child lying to you.

Have you ever noticed that you don't tend to get hungry when you're busy and then, when you start thinking about food, suddenly you want it? There's a fundamental relationship between thinking about food and eating. When you're craving food even when you aren't hungry, it's likely that you're bored, tired, stressed, or trying to avoid something you don't want to do. You're probably looking for a way to distract yourself from the resistance you're feeling and the negative or stressful thoughts that underlie it.

These thoughts create uncomfortable feelings, and rather than ignore them or sit with them until they dissipate, you make a beeline to the refrigerator to change your experience. Yet when something happens that requires your immediate attention, food is the farthest thing from your mind. When the house is on fire, I guarantee that you're not thinking about your stomach. If you're thinking about food when you aren't hungry, try asking yourself, "What experience am I trying to avoid right now?"

The problem with thinking about food is that it leads to eating. Of course, this isn't a problem if you're actually hungry and it's time to eat. But if you're in the habit of thinking about food often, it's likely that you're eating more food, and more pleasure food in particular, than your body needs. Thinking about food can become our mind's default position, coming in whenever we're stressed, excited, overwhelmed, upset, elated, or bored—any excuse to think about food will do. The key to skinny thinking is becoming more aware of how you think about food and how often you think about it.

Seeing the Whole Picture

When we give in to a food craving, overeat junk food, or eat when we're not hungry, we're focusing on one thing—immediate pleasure. Seduced by the promise of pleasure, short-lived though it may be, we don't think about the not-so-nice consequences of our choice. Caught in magical thinking, we pretend that eating pleasure food will give us only what we want—relief and happiness—and nothing that we don't want.

We didn't create this habit on our own. Food advertising that stresses taste over health is aimed at the pleasure-seeking part of us and encourages the Child's way of thinking. It's a myopic perspective that zeroes in on a small sliver of truth about food—that it often tastes good. Bombarded each day by hundreds of messages about the taste of pleasure food, it's no wonder that our first impulse is to reach for it when we don't like whatever we're experiencing. While pleasure foods in small doses are fine, when they're the cornerstone of our diet, they're costly to our health.

Look at the table called "Consequences of Overeating and Following a Food Craving When You're Not Hungry" on page 25 that shows you the whole picture of food. Then close your eyes and imagine overeating a pleasure food when you're not hungry. What are the costs and benefits of this choice? We've already established that the Child tempts you by getting you to fantasize about tasting something delicious. But she doesn't tell you about the negative consequences of indulging a pleasure food craving when you're already full.

Overeating when your stomach is full requires a degree of self-delusion. In these moments, the Child is in charge because you're considering only taste, not health. You're thinking, "This tastes really nice. I want more of it, even though I'm full." To keep eating when you're full, you have to put blinders on and be willing to see only part of the truth, be willing to say to yourself, "Right now, I'm more interested in immediate gratification than any negative longer-term consequences."

Look at the table again. Really take it in. Create a mental snapshot of it and practice bringing it to mind repeatedly so that the next time the Child comes on the scene, you can counter her pleadings with a mental image of this table. You can then say, "Hold on a minute. You're not telling me the whole truth, that in exchange for spending a few short seconds with a pleasure food, I'll suffer for hours, days, or even weeks. That's a lousy trade-off. It's not worth it."

Next, take a look at the table entitled "Consequences of Eating Nutritious Food When You're Hungry" on page 26. Notice the long list of positive consequences of eating mostly nutritious food. What a radical departure from the first table! This is the whole picture of changing your diet and eating healthily. Take a mental snapshot of this table as well. When you have an opportunity to choose between eating pleasure food and eating nutritiously, remember your mental images of these tables.

Consequences of Overeating and Following a
Food Craving When You're Not Hungry

Positive Consequences	Negative Consequences
We taste something that we like.	The taste only lasts for a short time.
We avoid feeling an uncomfortable feeling for the moment.	The taste leads to wanting to taste more and eat more.
	We feel guilty for eating a food that is caloric and not nutritious.
	We feel guilty for overeating.
	We berate ourselves for not having enough willpower.
	We gain weight.
	We undercut our growth by not discovering the beliefs that are generating our uncomfortable emotions.
	We hide because we feel too fat and can't fit into our clothes.
	We lose confidence professionally and socially.
	We feel physically uncomfortable: bloated, nauseated, or listless.

Consequences of Eating Nutritious Food When You're Hungry

Positive Consequences	Negative Consequences
Our taste buds readjust.	We occasionally miss the taste of junk.
We come to like the taste of nutritious food.	
We feel proud of ourselves for eating healthfully.	
We gain confidence because we're treating ourselves better.	
We lose the urge to binge and we regain our power over food.	
We become healthier and more energetic.	
We set a good example for others.	
We stop eating emotionally as a result of using inquiry to examine our beliefs.	
Our body reaches and stabilizes at a healthy weight.	

Worshipping the Golden Calf

During Moses's absence, when he was climbing Mount Sinai, the Israelites cast an enormous statue of a golden calf. Imagining that it contained supernatural powers, they laid offerings at its feet and prayed to it for miracles.

When Moses returned, he was incensed that the children of Israel, believers in the one God, had reverted to pagan behavior. Resolving to put an end to it, he implored his fellow Jews to stop this foolish practice, and to notice that their statue was inert and undeserving of the powers and status they had bestowed upon it.

Moses asked his brethren how a statue they had created with their own hands could possibly be God. How could it have the power to remove their heartaches or grant their prayers? In this way, Moses helped the Israelites to see that they had been engaged in magical thinking.

Hearing this story, it's easy to poke fun at the Israelites and label their behavior as ignorant or even comical. How could they have been so foolish as to mistake an idol for God? Yet when we install food on our altars, and view it as our God, companion, and savior, we are no different! The Israelites expected a metal calf to provide them with what it could not just as we look to food to give *us* what it cannot.

"Simple enough," you may say. But how do you break the habit of turning to food in your time of need or celebration or longing? The answer is: Take another look. Open yourself to a broader perspective and come to see the whole truth about food rather than just hanging on to your habitual, unquestioned assumptions.

Granted, not wanting what you think you want is a tricky business, because in your moment of wanting, nothing seems clearer or more powerful than your desire. In those moments, the Child is powerful; she has your undivided attention and it takes tremendous will to say, "Not now, dear, maybe later," just as you might to a child who wants a snack right before dinner.

Listening to and following the dictates of the Child is a habit that has grown stronger through years of repetition and reinforcement. But if you believe that breaking this habit is daunting, just remember—you created it in the first place, so you have the power to uncreate it.

Of course, the ego wants you to view the desire to experience the taste pleasure of food as impossible to resist because that keeps you from challenging the ego's authority. But now is the time to let go of this false story that you've created.

My own favorite fiction was that the almighty hold that food had over me was a dastardly plan created by God to keep me suffering and struggling. And, of course, because God created it, I was powerless to thwart it. To break free, I had to realize that I was the kingmaker and had the power to debunk my story and withdraw my misguided projection. The power of choice had always rested in me and once I accepted that, I chose to dethrone food by changing the way I thought about it.

If the Child is tempting you with pleasure food and you're not hungry, ask yourself: "What am I telling myself that's creating the impulse to reach for food? What am I thinking? What am I feeling right now?" Then ask yourself if eating the pleasure food will truly satisfy that impulse. Will it alleviate the feeling? Will it solve the problem that you're ruminating over? Will it rewrite history or alleviate worries about the future? Will it allow you to say the things you wanted to say in that conversation with your coworker or spouse or child? What will two minutes with that particular food give you? Are the negative consequences of shame, blame, self-castigation, lethargy, ill health, and weight gain worth it?

For those of us with eating and weight issues, food has been our golden calf. But once we've seen the whole truth about food, we can't believe in it or idolize it in the same way. This inexorably changes us and sets the stage for a new, pragmatic, rational relationship with food. It's time to melt down your golden calf and see food for what it always has been—not a god—just food with a lowercase "f."

What Story Are You In?

If you notice an urge to eat something when you're not hungry, you're probably involved in a story—something negative that the mind is telling you about yourself, life, others, or something you're doing. At those moments, you're arguing with reality, resisting the way life is showing up. Some examples of typical stories you may be running prior to an urge to attack the cookie jar are:

- ✹ I'm bored.
- ✹ I don't want to do this project.
- ✹ I screwed things up again.

⊛ I don't want to make this phone call that I'm supposed to make.
⊛ I hate filing.
⊛ I can't face the piles of work on my desk.
⊛ Time to balance my checkbook again.

When you're resisting the task in front of you, the idea of distracting yourself with an exciting taste experience can be tempting. A vision of hot fudge cascading down slopes of pure white vanilla ice cream can transport us from the monotony of daily life. Who couldn't use a respite from changing the sheets or preparing the taxes or any other task we love to avoid? The habit of eating pleasure food to change our experience, to escape and entertain ourselves rather than nourish our bodies, is an innocent way of trying to love and soothe ourselves when we're bored or under stress. There's no reason to make ourselves feel bad or wrong about this.

However, overfilling our tank has consequences that don't feel loving, like indigestion, lethargy, or feeling bloated, nauseated, headachy, or sleepy. We may feel guilty, regretful, or angry, and judge ourselves for lacking willpower when we gain weight and our clothes feel tight.

What's a girl to do? First, if you notice your hand reaching toward the cookie jar or the ice cream in the freezer when you're full, walk into another room, away from the food and ask, "What story am I in?" or "What am I believing that's not true?" or "What do I really need right now?" Get quiet and take a few minutes with these questions. Almost always, you will find a painful emotion or some unease lurking underneath this impulse.

One of the costs of overindulging in pleasure food is that it prevents you from experiencing or inquiring about what you're feeling or believing that caused you to want to eat. The Child goes after pleasure as a way of coping with what it doesn't like about life. When you automatically indulge and fulfill a desire, you miss out on its real message: There's something that's off here that I need to address, either inside myself, in my life, or with another person. Keep this in mind and notice when the Child starts talking to you. Ask yourself, "Is there something that I'm resisting about life, something that I'm trying to cope with by seeking pleasure? Why do I need pleasure now? What do I really need?"

Inquiry: Is It True?

After you've uncovered the belief or story that caused you to feel bad and want to overeat, like a good prosecutor, begin to gather evidence to support the veracity of your belief. Is the story you're telling yourself true? If you're going to believe something and let it ruin your mood and run your life, shouldn't it at least be true? As a reasonable, rational adult, shouldn't that be your minimum requirement?

When you are tied up in a negative story, like the ones listed in the previous section, ask yourself, "Can I absolutely know that this is true? Can I know that I shouldn't have to do this task? Is it really true that I'm always making a mess of things or that so-and-so is always busting my chops?"

I've discovered that my painful beliefs are big fat lies or, at the very least, partial truths. It's been amazing to see that those beliefs that caused me to overeat and feel bad may have contained only a sliver of truth, but that the ego used that sliver to hook me. And, gosh darn it! I'd been living and punishing myself with them as if they were gospel! Thankfully, when you see that you've been suckered—really see it—you become liberated from those beliefs. If they arise again, you can notice them, and flick them away like you would a mosquito.

How We Delude Ourselves about Food

Two Sides of the Desire Coin

Slow down and notice what happens during a meal. When you first sit down, assuming you're hungry, the first few bites taste delicious. But as you move toward satiation, the experience changes, the law of diminishing returns sets in, and each successive bite becomes less pleasurable. Once you're satiated, the pleasure drops off even faster, until each additional bite becomes downright unpleasant!

Eating pleasure food has a tendency to turn into overeating pleasure food. One of the characteristics of pleasure food is that it tastes so darn good that it's hard to stop eating it. How can you be expected to resist eating more of something that was designed to be irresistible? Even when you're stuffed and your stomach is groaning, you still want to taste more. We delude ourselves into thinking that if we continue eating, we can squeeze a bit more pleasure out of the experience, but alas, all we get is pain.

The human impulse to hold on to pleasure and avoid pain is an important part of the whole picture of food. But we live in a world where desire is governed by duality, and overindulging in pleasure is inexorably linked to pain. Just like trying to separate two sides of a coin, you can't peel the pleasure away from the pain.

An Affair to Remember

We have such a hard time resisting pleasure food because of the emotional attachment we formed with it in childhood. In this section, I'll take you back to my romantic beginnings with food. As you read, travel back to how you first formed an emotional connection with food.

Butter was big in our family. When margarine came into fashion, Mom was quick to tell us that she couldn't see giving up the flavor of butter, despite the health consequences of eating it. But I don't ever remember seeing her eat it. She was very thin.

My Grandma Helen, on the other hand, was a butter sneaker. She was a fun-loving woman who used to eat butter straight off the knife when she thought no one was looking. She came over on a boat from Russia when she was an infant, and Mom said her butter sneaking was the peasant in her that was never bred out. For me, the takeaway message was that eating rich foods like butter was low class.

Mom used to tell me stories about when she was a teenager and went to dinners at her Aunt Ruth's house. Ruth was a willowy fashionista who always slathered a thick layer of butter on Mom's bread before serving it to her. Even though she hardly ate anything herself, Ruth put lots of food on other people's plates—apparently enjoying the thrill of eating vicariously. I concluded that fashionable, thin women fed butter to others, but didn't actually eat it themselves.

Chocolate-related matters were unequivocally my father's domain. He was our family's resident chocoholic. Chocolate ice cream, marshmallow sauce, hot fudge, and peanuts were staples in our household. Every night, our after-dinner ritual was doling out massive slabs of chocolate ice cream. On the weekends, it was root beer floats and chocolate milkshakes a la Dad.

We ate so much chocolate ice cream that Dad, silver-tongued devil that he was, convinced the fountain manager at the local Thrifty store to sell it to us in bulk. I remember accompanying him on his bimonthly treks to Thrifty and hefting three-gallon commercial tubs into the car, then depositing them in our second freezer (devoted entirely to ice cream, of course). Unbeknownst to him, Dad was validating my burgeoning chocolate fetish, letting me know by example that eating lots and lots of chocolate was perfectly fine, even normal.

We ate mountains of chocolate ice cream every night while watching Hawaii Five-O *or* All in the Family. *Although my mom's portions were the same size as ours, she nursed hers, letting it melt into brown soup, which she eventually poured down the sink. For my mother, my model of womanhood, rich food was something to have around but not eat. Yet I found myself unable to follow her example; if it was there, I ate it.*

I remember chocolate being a big part of my life even as early as age four. Once, knowing that my parents kept M&M's in the cabinet over the washer, I dragged a chair over, climbed up, and reached for the bag. The next thing I knew, I was being hoisted off the washer, smacked on the bottom, and promptly sent to my room.

As I got older, every day when I came home for lunch, a full cup of Nestlé chocolate chips awaited me for dessert. It was given to me, I thought, as a reward for spending my morning at school, away from home and family. As a result, I began to see chocolate as a treat and associated it with feeling loved and accepted. As I got older, when I felt upset, I would zone out in front of the television with a bowl of chocolate ice cream. Somehow, because whatever was bothering me faded into the background, I came to associate sweets with the experience of comfort and relief. Little did I know that I was sowing the seeds for relating to food as a friend rather than as sustenance.

Our Relationship with Food

Food tantalizes our senses, beckoning us with mouthwatering aromas and titillating tastes and textures. That, compounded by the fact that human beings are programmed to love food, makes for a perfect storm for an overeating and weight-control disaster. Eating is pleasurable, and there's nothing wrong with enjoying food. Yet when food becomes the object of our desire, our secret passion, entertainment, or a naughty indulgence, we've turned it into something it's not—a lover.

Unconsciously, we can imbue food with the power to fill many physical and emotional needs. It becomes our ideal friend and lover who is always available, never lets us down, never puts us down, and never says no. Epitomizing fidelity, no matter what is happening in our lives, whether we feel on top of the world or down in the dumps, food is there to keep us company. For the fleeting moment it spends in our mouth, our favorite food always delivers.

Ultimately, healing means withdrawing our romantic projections, seeing food as nice-tasting nutrition, not the stuff that we can't wait to curl up with and get into our mouths. Rather than "Oh, sweet brownie, how I love you and long to taste your rich, chocolaty goodness," our food thoughts might sound like "I'm hungry and it's time to eat. What will I have? My body could use some protein and vegetables. I have X in the house, so I will create Y meal." Although it may not be sexy or exciting, this new way of thinking sets the stage for a healthy, rational, mature relationship with food.

Pleasure

If you eat for pleasure, chances are that you see food as your friend, a treat, or a reward rather than just as nourishment. It's a very deeply embedded view in which food becomes larger than life, taking on a glorified and revered position in your life. You blow its importance out of proportion relative to what it can actually offer you. Because you see your relationship with pleasure food as more important to your happiness than it truly is, if you allow yourself to eat it after abstaining from it on a diet, you can easily go hog wild.

But it's important to notice that the pleasure from eating is fleeting! Soon after you put something in your mouth, the experience of eating is over. That's part of the whole truth that the Child doesn't want you to know. It can be liberating to realize that if you don't have two minutes with a particular food, it really won't impact your life.

When we habitually think about food in a way that creates excitement and pleasurable sensations, it makes food seem wonderfully fun and special, and this can leave us in an emotionally charged trance of sorts. Without realizing it, we slip into another state of consciousness, where seeing the whole truth about food is impossible. Once we realize how untrue and overblown our thinking is about it, we're well on our way to thinking about it differently.

Glorifying food is a habit of believing that we need it to be happy and to feel good. But we don't. As we examine our beliefs about food and discover the truth, we realize that we never needed to get pleasure from food because life itself is pleasurable.

The Truth about Loving Food

The truth about loving food is that at a certain point, it stops loving you back. Actually, that isn't even true. Food can't love you back. Food is just food. It's fuel that gives the body energy to go about its business. But it's fuel that tastes good and is pleasurable to eat, and that's an undeniable part of the eating equation.

With so many other pleasures available, why have so many of us become fixated on and addicted to food? What's its allure? I'd wager that most would say that food captures our hearts and imaginations because it looks, smells, and tastes so good. It activates all five of our senses. From the moment that we lift food-laden forks to our lips, there is no denying the pleasure it gives us. Or is there? Are we totally sure about this pleasure assumption?

Ask any of us who have been overly involved with food, who have spent countless waking hours thinking and dreaming about, salivating over, and anticipating our next meal, and we would swear that food is our favorite thing in the universe. We would passionately argue that the experience of eating trumps most other pleasures.

But if you're nodding away at that statement like an enthusiastic bobblehead toy, then answer this question: When was the last time you *just* ate while you were eating? When was the last time you ate without watching television, listening to the radio, reading, driving, or having a conversation? When, of your own volition, did you just eat without any other add-on experiences?

Now, imagine eating your favorite food all by yourself with no other distractions. Does this sound appealing? If not, why not?

If food were truly the love of your life, why would you need to couple eating with other activities? Why isn't eating, this so-called most pleasurable experience, enough? Hmm? Maybe, just maybe, your idea of eating doesn't match up to the truth about it. Maybe you haven't been seeing the whole truth about food.

There is no denying that while food is in our mouths, it tastes good. Yet prolonging the pleasure means inserting more and more food. And if we do this, we all know what happens. When we follow one bite with another and end up overfilling our stomachs, in no time, the experience of eating shifts into something else. The pleasure turns into pain. The excited anticipation turns into aversion.

The truth about loving food is that it tastes good for only a short while and if we try to draw out its taste pleasure, our love soon turns to hate, and weight gain, guilt, self-castigation, lethargy, and aversion follow in quick succession. Does it really make sense to romanticize an experience when the pleasure you derive from it is so fleeting? Or are there other ways you can take care of yourself that are *truly* fulfilling and nurturing? Ask yourself, "How can I feed my soul and experience the kind of joy that can't fade or turn into its opposite?"

The Pleasure Scale

Imagine a pleasure scale that goes from 1 to 10, with 10 being the most pleasurable experience you can imagine. A "1" might be brushing your teeth or combing your hair and a "10" might be an epiphany, great sex, connecting with a close friend, or, for food lovers, that first bite of a favorite food.

Before reading on (don't peek), take a moment and list your other, nonfood "9's" and "10's" on a sheet of paper or in your journal.

An important part of withdrawing your romanticization of food is finding other activities that are pleasurable and meaningful. What are other "10's" for you? What do you enjoy that doesn't bring the suffering that accompanies your all-consuming love affair with food? Food may never become a "1" for you, but hopefully, after practicing the Five Steps, you will be able to see it as a "5" or a "6."

Here are some "9's" and "10's" that my workshop participants have shared with me:

- Being totally engaged in what you're doing
- Feeling a heart connection with someone
- Being in nature
- Giving
- Being of service
- Being aligned with my true self
- Reading a great book
- Reaching orgasm

- Hugging and cuddling
- Sitting by the ocean
- Looking into the eyes of a pet
- Looking into the eyes of someone I love
- Feeling seen
- Accomplishing something I didn't think I could do
- Singing
- Watching a good movie
- Making music
- Dancing
- Making art
- Laughing
- Reaching a goal
- Exceeding someone's expectations
- Living my life's purpose
- Doing meaningful work
- Walking around on a beautiful day
- Having a massage
- Taking a bubble bath
- Lifting someone's spirit when he or she is down

Letting Go of Romanticizing Food

Part of our healing requires us to stop glamorizing food by withdrawing some of our false projections onto it and false meanings we've given to it. A balanced relationship with food would be more like your relationship with toilet paper. Okay, I admit this is a crude analogy, but with both food and toilet paper, quality is important. They both fill a need (when you need it, you need it!), the experience of using them is quick, and most importantly, there's no need to think about them when you're not using them. It's not like you're going to create an overblown fantasy anticipating the velvety softness of two-ply Cottonelle!

Take a moment now to notice any romantic thoughts you might have about food and ask if these projections are really true. Can food fulfill you and give you lasting pleasure?

When you go without food and don't think about it, you see the truth: You really don't need food as a source of pleasure. Of course, you need it to survive, but you don't need to have a certain food at a particular time. When you don't think about food, you're free of it, and you see that you don't need to have a romance with it. Then, your relationship with it can become very practical and healthy.

Instead of dreaming about food like you might fantasize about sex, notice the pleasure in being alive, in performing simple everyday tasks, and in thinking about food in a practical way. The romantic relationship disappears as you see the complete truth about what food can and can't offer you. The way we think about food is the crux of our problems with it. If our romanticization of and longing for food go away, then our problem with food goes away.

Feelings

Where Feelings Come From

Feelings manifest as sensations in the body, making them seem much more real than thoughts. If we feel a certain way, that feeling must be true, right? As if this weren't enough, inflated by self-righteousness, the ego comes up with all the reasons why *we're right* about our feelings, feeding a given emotion with more thoughts, pumping it up until it achieves its desired objective—action. The ego is always looking for a fight, and the worse we feel, the better it likes it.

Feelings come from thoughts. It seems like this should be common knowledge, found in a standard-issue operating manual on how to live as a human being. Just think—if we had known that feelings come from thoughts when we were children, we could have learned to deal with our stressful thoughts by either ignoring or questioning them. In fact, we could have avoided creating negative feelings in the first place!

Maintaining our emotional hygiene by debunking negative thoughts would have become second nature—the only sane way to live. Unpleasant emotions would have been rare once we understood that we had the power to stop creating them. When a stressful belief arose, we would have been able to catch it and say to ourselves, "Oh, that's just conditioning," and ignore it. If we bought into a belief and accidentally created a negative feeling, an alarm bell would have sounded inside us and immediately we would have asked, "What am I believing right now that's causing me to feel this way?" That question would have yanked us out of the ego and transported us back to the rational, pleasant world of the true self.

But we didn't learn these things as children, and so we've become accustomed to listening to and believing stressful thoughts that create anger, sadness, and fear. With practice, though, we can still learn to catch feelings before they form. We have a choice. We don't have to travel the well-trodden path of letting negative thoughts generate negative feelings. Instead, we can form a new habit of ignoring the egoic mind and seeing thoughts as simply results of our conditioning.

One reason our feelings feel so real and overwhelming is that we identify or merge with them. We become the anger or sadness or fear. We think that it's *our* anger and feel self-righteous about it: "It's mine, and I have a right to express it, and you'd better respect it!"

But who says that feelings belong to us? Or even that thoughts belong to us? Both arise and subside unbidden. If we feel ownership of our emotions and believe they're meaningful, it will be harder to let them arise and subside naturally. We'll want to hold on to them, feel their power, and feed them with more thoughts and beliefs that justify their presence. Then, we'll want others to validate our position and our right to feel what we feel.

Instead, if we can remember that we are *that which is aware* of emotion, rather than the emotion itself, it will have far less power over us. From this vantage point, we can watch the action without getting involved in it. For example, anger happens. It arises, it's felt, it does its dance, it subsides—and we remain unchanged. We are only the space in which anger arises and are completely unsullied by it.

Anger, Stress, and Other Arguments with Reality

Anger is the Critic saying to life, "Oh, no you didn't." It has always been my issue. Life never happens fast enough for me and people don't quite do or say what I expect them to. Almost always there is a disparity between what I want and what is actually happening. And boom— there's anger!

Stress, on the other hand, is how we put a nice face on anger. It's anger in disguise. It's the ego getting mad at life, God, and whoever else is around, saying, "This is too much. Life feels overwhelming. I don't have enough time or energy to do all of this!"

Stress really kicks up for me when two or more people ask me to do things at the same time. The people pleaser in me freaks out because I know that I'm going to disappoint someone. I'm convinced that this is a no-win situation. Someone will probably get upset with me, and that notion alone will upset me. I'm frantically searching for the escape hatch—anything that will get me out of there. Of course, the Child has an easy answer—reach for something yummy to eat.

Whenever we're upset about what's happening, we're arguing with reality. Life in the form of a particular situation has already happened. It's a fact, and there's nothing we can do about it. As author Byron Katie says, "When we fight with life we lose, but only 100% of the time!" Our resistance to life is created by the thought "This shouldn't be happening." This is the most common way that we cause our own suffering.

Whenever we're irritated by a situation—we're waiting in a traffic jam or someone breaks a promise—the mind tends to jump in and proclaim that this or that *should* be different: "There *should* be more staff on the cash registers so that people don't have to wait for such a long time"; "They *shouldn't* make a promise they can't keep"; "They *should* have known better"; "This slow car in front of me *should* go faster."

Notice what happens when you use the word "should." There's an immediate contraction in your body. You're resisting life and that doesn't feel good. Your perspective narrows down to a tiny sliver of the truth about a situation and you miss seeing the whole picture. Seeing only the reasons why things *should* be different, you don't consider the possible benefits of the situation.

When we're standing in a long checkout line at the supermarket, we don't consider the possibility that waiting provides an opportunity for quiet contemplation. The broken promise gives us a chance to learn discernment: seeing whom we can depend on. By remembering how it felt when we made a promise that we didn't keep, we're able to sidestep judgment and learn compassion and forgiveness, instead. Here are some other ways to respond to an unexpected or unwelcome situation:

1. *You can look at the potential benefit that comes with this new development.* You don't have to jump right to the downside or what you think *should* be happening, as you might have done in the past. Considering the benefit eliminates the reaction altogether. Don't be discouraged if it takes a lot of practice to get to this point.

2. *You can recognize that your conditioning is coming up in the form of anger and say, "Oh, that's just my conditioning."* This noticing helps you dis-identify with your negative story and let it go. If you're quick enough, you'll notice and dis-identify with it before the anger or stress has a chance to erupt in your body!

3. *If you miss your chance in #2, notice and acknowledge that you've been triggered.* You can say something like, "Wow, I've really been triggered" or "I'm really in reaction." Noticing and telling yourself the truth brings you back to the present moment, takes you out of the story you're running and into the Wise Witness.

4. *Be gentle with yourself and let it be okay that you're in reaction.* Ironically, this will move you into acceptance! Once you're in acceptance, even if you found it by accepting the fact that you're in resistance, you can go back to your true self!

When we were young, many of us who now suffer from addictions were terrified of anger. Because grown-ups looked enormous, we were afraid that if they got angry enough, they would hurt or even kill us. Unconsciously, we believed that if we provoked others or allowed ourselves to feel intense anger, we would either be killed or our rage would be so out of control that we would kill others. Associating anger with death, we avoided these emotions at all costs and numbed out with food (or some other substance) instead.

Depression

If there were a hit parade of the top reasons for overeating, anger, depression, and sadness would be right up there, along with boredom. If depression had a voice, it would say, "Everything is hopeless. What's the point of living?" Its energy is deadly, obliterating every ray of hope in its path.

For the ego, the way out of depression is to distract itself with immediate pleasure. The Child says, "The only thing that would make me feel halfway decent is food. What do I have to lose anyway?" So, reaching for food when depression strikes becomes as predictable as the sun rising each morning. After all, stuffing your depression with sexy pleasure food is the path of least resistance. But you know what it has to offer: a fleeting, nice taste in your mouth and hell to pay afterwards.

The question is how do you turn this pattern around? We've come to believe that when the Child comes on the scene, we have no choice but to listen and follow her directions. The truth, though, is that the past is *not* a reliable predictor of the future. Just because you've reached for food 620,000 times before doesn't mean you have to do it now. You can choose health over your conditioning, your true self over the ego.

Rather than listening to the Child coaxing you down a self-destructive road to food hell, ask yourself if you're willing to try something different. Just this once, are you willing to stop the action and not reach for food? Instead of stuffing down the depression or sadness with food, could you allow it to be present and ask yourself, "What story am I in right now? What am I believing that's causing me to feel flattened and down on myself and life?" You can even tell the Child that she can still eat later, if that's what she wants, but not right now. The next time depression or sadness is on the scene, try this experiment and see what happens.

Boredom

When we're bored, we tell ourselves the unhappy story that whatever is happening is uninteresting and not what we were hoping for from life. We feel restless and dissatisfied. The ego doesn't like what's showing up, yet it has no clarity about how to remedy it. Boredom is a muddled, stuck state that the ego creates, agonizes over, and turns into a problem. Oftentimes, when we tell ourselves a story that results in boredom, we move into default mode—reaching for something tasty. We allow the Child to take over, and see food solely as a source of pleasure. One way to avoid reaching for food when boredom strikes is to say to the Child, just as we might to a persistent two-year-old, "Not now—maybe later."

The Wise Witness remembers the whole truth about pleasure food, that even though it may taste nice for a few fleeting seconds, it can't alleviate boredom. If we eat it and we're not hungry, it may not taste as good as we had imagined or we may overeat it and end up feeling worse because we gave into our craving. Seeing the whole truth about food from the perspective of the Wise Witness interrupts the automatic tendency to reach for food when we're bored.

The other point to remember is that when we eat to numb out, we miss the opportunity to heal whatever conditioning is arising. The next time you're bored, ask yourself "What is my true self's experience of boredom?" You know the ego's experience, but become aware of how your true self *just notices* the boredom. It isn't the generator of the feeling (the ego is), and it isn't affected by it either. It just notices boredom arising and doesn't evaluate it as something to like or not like. It isn't trying to get life to conform to a certain feeling. It's just humming along, okay with everything as it is.

When boredom arises, we can become aware of it and realize that it's not who we really are. In other words, we can dis-identify with it. Who we are is able to notice the ego being bored. We can simply allow the feeling of boredom to be present and reengage in what we're doing. When we allow a negative feeling to be present without trying to make it dissipate or when we're fully engaged in what we're doing, we're not thinking. And if we're not thinking, we automatically align with our true self and we can't be bored. What a blessing!

Fear and Worry

At their core, fear and worry are about survival. They are the equivalent of the ego lamenting, "This looks bad. I don't know if I'm going to make it." Even when the ego is worried about other people, ultimately, it's still afraid for itself. "If something happens to them, then what will I do? How will I get along?"

Excitement and happiness can even lead us to reach for food, because fear of loss is usually lurking somewhere underneath, generated by thoughts like "This will never last"; "What will happen when they leave?"; or "Just wait, they'll find out you're a fraud soon enough."

The egoic mind invents a scary future and we're instantly trapped in fear's clutches. I've heard that 90% of the things we fear never happen. If you look at it from that perspective, why are we getting ourselves all worked up? Who knows what the future will bring? Why get our knickers in a bunch about a nightmare that in all likelihood will never manifest?

Worrying is a habit born out of the desire to be in control. The ego keeps busy trying to convince you that you can bend life to your will if you live by the ego's rules. And when life has the audacity to say "Thanks, but no thanks" to the ego's plan, the ego wigs out and says, "Holy cannoli! I'm just a fragile little speck in this vast, unfriendly universe. Who will take care of me? I'll never be safe!" Then, before you can say "all-you-can-eat buffet," in bolts the Child to comfort you, assuring you, "You know what you can always depend on, what never lets you down? Your good old friend food. There are no surprises in that relationship. You always know what you're going to get when you bite into an apple fritter or a slice of pizza."

Just because fear and worry arise doesn't mean we have to avoid them through food. They can't hurt us and like all other feelings, they eventually dissipate. We can allow them to be present and learn to tolerate them after all. The best way to deal with fear and worry is to ask, "What's the worst thing that could happen?" Once we realize that, even if the worst thing happens, we can deal with it.

Slow Down the Action

One important step in dealing with feelings is to *slow down the action*. This can be challenging because addictive patterns make us go into "zombie" mode, distracting us and keeping us from being present in the moment.

Set the intention and ask for help from the Wise Witness to *be present* when an eating compulsion strikes. By setting this intention, you commit to your own healing and plant your feet squarely on Recovery Road. It's as if you're saying, "I'm ready to move on and transform my dysfunctional relationship with food."

After you've set the intention, even if you continue to go unconscious the next 20, 50, or 500 times the impulse to eat comes up, something in you will remember that intention, and eventually you'll be able to interrupt the emotional food-stuffing response. The more often you can interrupt your usual pattern, the easier it will become. Just as you created the old habit of eating in response to frightening and uncomfortable emotions, you can create a new habit of awareness by slowing down the action and removing yourself from the danger zone—wherever the food is.

Eating When You're Not Hungry

Anatomy of a Craving

A craving is an overwhelming desire for a particular food that screams for immediate fulfillment. Memories of eating a pleasure food entice us to want to taste it again and, voila, a craving is born. When a craving strikes, it takes over and becomes all we can think about. Not fulfilling the craving isn't even an option. The issue is not if we can have the object of our desire, but when.

When a craving is on the scene, it can feel like it's driving and we're just along for the ride. When we finally fulfill our desire, finally bite into that donut or piece of chocolate cake, we *credit the food* for the momentary bliss we feel.

But we have it backwards. *It's the craving that caused the suffering*, not our being deprived of the object of our desire. And *it's the elimination of the craving that caused the bliss,* not the food. We feel great because we're no longer burdened by the craving, yet we mistakenly give the credit to the chocolate cake.

If we overeat the chocolate cake, the suffering isn't really gone, but transformed into the guilt and self-loathing we feel after indulging. The ego keeps our thinking compartmentalized so that in the throes of a craving, we think only about the object of our desire, not the complete experience. We become the Scarlett O'Haras of eating, opining, "I'll think about that tomorrow." This is how we dupe ourselves into indulging and suffering again and again. We think only about the fleeting pleasure we get from fulfilling the craving and ignore the negative repercussions. Here's the ego's version of following a craving versus the complete experience:

The Ego's Version: *Craving → Obtaining the Object of Desire → Fulfillment*

The Complete Experience: *Craving → Indulgence → Momentary Pleasure Due to Elimination of the Desire → Guilt, Self-Loathing, and Weight Gain*

The other way we fool ourselves when a craving hits is to tell ourselves that we can have just a little of what we desire and then stop. But if we're addicted to a food, it's very difficult to stick to that plan. Most of us end up overeating because we don't find the satisfaction we expect, and there's no clear signal to stop other than the pain of an overstuffed belly.

If we could eat just a little of something we crave, we wouldn't suffer the physical, emotional, and spiritual consequences that often go hand in hand with addictive pleasures. We would break the cycle and take our power back. Unfortunately, most people with food issues can't do this.

The Child

When you hear that familiar voice inside your head demanding "I want to eat this now," you can be sure the Child is on the scene. On the other hand, the wise adult part of us wants to eat a particular food because it's part of our nutritional agenda for the day. The Child gets us into trouble, and the more we can recognize her, the less power she has over us. Every time we decide not to respond to her, we reduce her power.

If we're very identified with the Child, however, it can feel like we have no choice with regard to her demands. They can feel like life or death imperatives. "Eat this now, not two minutes from now," she says. "I want it now. Let me have it. I'll hate you if you don't give it to me."

The Child rationalizes, plays games, and hooks us with partial truths about food that have nothing to do with its nutrition (the real reason we eat it), focusing on pleasure, not what the body actually needs. Unconcerned about what's good or bad for her, she just wants what she wants and doesn't see the consequences of fulfilling her desires in the way an adult would.

The more you can recognize the Child aspect of yourself, the easier it will be to align with the Wise Witness and take your power back. The Wise Witness knows there's a price to pay for following this pleasure-seeking principle, and if you strengthen your Wise Witness by listening to it more, you will feel less compelled to follow the dictates of the Child.

There's no need to be rigid about this. When the desire to eat pleasure food arises, just recognize it: "Oh, that's the Child." Doing this lessens the Child's power because, all of a sudden, you realize that what you thought you wanted is really just what the Child wants. In seeing this, you've dis-identified with the Child. When you see the truth, it interrupts the pattern and cuts through it.

The two benefits of dis-identifying with the Child are that it weakens the ego and leaves you with time to make a more rational choice. Instead of indulging, you might say, "I'm not going to indulge the Child right now." Or, like a wise parent, you might just say no: "No, you can't have another cookie." Or, from a place of choice and detachment, you might decide, "Okay, let's have some pleasure." In that case, you're choosing rather than reacting based on compulsion.

When you react out of habit, it feels like you have no choice. But when you're aligned with the Wise Witness, you're free to make a choice. When you're listening to and obeying the Child, you're bound. That's a huge difference! The goal is to recognize that you're not the Child and develop enough distance from her so that you're free from unconsciously acquiescing to her and indulging her demands.

When you see that the "I" that craves is the ego and *not you*, it is much easier to ignore a craving. You become *that which is noticing the Child craving food*. From that place of dis-identification, you can turn your attention elsewhere. Don't be discouraged if, in the beginning, your noticing is still followed by eating. The pattern of following your thoughts into the kitchen may be deeply entrenched. Fortunately, if you're patient and vigilant, noticing these food thoughts will eventually lead to being able to ignore them.

Kung Fu for Cravings and Emotional Eating

Have you ever had a feeling of gnawing, insatiable emptiness that just won't let go of you? That is what I felt when I was on the verge of an emotional-eating attack. Something or someone was bugging me, and all I wanted to do was stuff myself with the best-tasting food I could find. I wasn't picky at that point. I just *needed* to eat something, pronto! This feeling of urgency was so strong because I'd followed it and reinforced it over and over for years.

Eating was how I coped with life. If life didn't feel good, I indulged in negative thoughts that made me feel even worse. To feel better, I ate too much. If stress or an uncomfortable emotion came on the scene, my hand automatically reached for food, and I turned into an eating machine. Happiness was the issue and eating a mere symptom.

Emotional eating is eating without being completely aware that you're eating. Instead, you're thinking and feeling—and feeding your feelings with—stressful thoughts while semi-consciously shoveling down copious quantities of food, perhaps without even tasting it.

If this has been your habit, the compulsion to eat feels so strong that it seems physical. The strength of the compulsion is actually due to the countless times you've reinforced it by reaching for food to soothe uncomfortable emotions. But fear not! It's possible to interrupt this pattern, and the following list of powerful kung fu exercises can help.

As you go through the list, think about your last emotional-eating attack. Then, imagine yourself using each kung fu as a sort of dress rehearsal, an opportunity to practice so the next time a craving or emotional-eating attack arises, you're ready. You'll have already used the tools.

Because different tools work better for different people, I've listed many kung fus. Your job is to go through them and *pick and practice one or two* that resonate with you. After a few fits and starts, I realized that kung fu #7 was tailor-made for me. I used it almost exclusively to break my emotional-eating habit. The key is to find a kung fu that's easy for you to remember under stress. You don't want to have to run and grab this book to jog your memory. Pretty soon, using your kung fu will become automatic and that habit will replace your old habit of emotional eating.

Powerful Kung Fu #1: Dis-identify with the Feeling

1. Notice that a craving is on the scene and get yourself the heck out of the kitchen!
2. Ask yourself, "What am I feeling right now?" Wait for the answer.
3. When the answer comes, ask yourself, "**What is noticing [the particular feeling you are feeling]?**" Fill in the blank with whatever feeling is present. Let's say agitation is present. Ask yourself, "What is noticing agitation?" This question helps you dis-identify with the feeling.

Or

Say to yourself, "**It's just [the particular feeling]. What a relief. It's not me. It couldn't be me because I'm over here, noticing it.**" It's such a huge relief to realize that the feeling is not you! Normally we merge with negative feelings and assume they're *our* feelings, but they belong to the ego, not to us—not to who we really are. When we identify with the feeling, we have little power or objectivity. But when we notice a feeling, we're outside of it, aligned with the Wise Witness. In my experience, this kung fu cuts the power of the feeling in half immediately.

Powerful Kung Fu #2: Allow the Feeling to Be There

1. Notice that a craving is on the scene and get yourself the heck out of the kitchen!

2. Drop your story about the feeling and simply allow it to be there. Notice the sensation. What does it feel like in your body? Allow the feeling to be there without any agenda for it to dissipate. Accepting it and allowing it to be present will enable it to eventually dissolve. Emotions don't come to stay; they come to leave. If you can learn to stop feeding them with more negative thoughts, they dissolve more quickly. The best internal posture is simply to be present and allow whatever is happening in the moment, without adding more negative thoughts to it. Ask yourself, **"Can I just allow [the particular feeling] to be there?"**

Powerful Kung Fu #3: Identify the Need

1. Notice that a craving is on the scene and get yourself the heck out of the kitchen!

2. Ask yourself, **"What am I needing right now that is causing me to want some pleasure?"**

3. If the answer is appreciation, comfort, or understanding, in your imagination, give yourself what you need—a hug or words of consolation or praise.

4. Alternatively, ask yourself, **"Is there something else here that's whole and complete and doesn't need anything?"** This will help you see the real you, the you that doesn't actually need what you may think you need.

Powerful Kung Fu #4: Is There Something I Need to Address?

1. Notice that a craving is on the scene and get yourself the heck out of the kitchen!

2. Ask yourself, **"Is there something I need to address inside myself, with another person, or in my life?"** Get curious about what that could be and be prepared for insights to arise. Then, take action to address any disharmonies or imbalances.

Powerful Kung Fu #5: Dis-identify with the Troublesome Food Thought

1. Notice that a craving is on the scene and get yourself the heck out of the kitchen!
2. Ask yourself, **"What is it that is aware of the thought 'I want food right now'?"**
3. Next, ask, **"Is that thought or impulse to eat really me? If I am aware of it, how can it be me?"** Once you realize that this thought is not you, you automatically dis-identify with it, and it loses its power.

Powerful Kung Fu #6: The Mosquito Flick

1. Notice that a craving is on the scene and get yourself the heck out of the kitchen!
2. Notice that an impractical food thought is on the scene and imagine flicking it away, the same way you would flick away an annoying mosquito.

Powerful Kung Fu #7: Notice that the Child Is on the Scene

1. Notice that a craving is on the scene and get yourself the heck out of the kitchen!
2. Tell yourself, **"Oh, that's just the Child. No big deal. For a minute there, I thought I wanted to eat something, but it was just what the Child wanted. She wanted to distract me. Thank goodness it's just the Child and not me."**

Powerful Kung Fu #8: See the Whole Picture of Food

1. Notice that a craving is on the scene and get yourself the heck out of the kitchen!
2. Remember the whole picture of food. The pleasure of eating a particular food is so short-lived! Imagine how bad you will feel if you overeat.

Powerful Kung Fu #9: Put Your Attention on Something Else

1. Notice that a craving is on the scene and get yourself the heck out of the kitchen!
2. Do or think about something else. Read a book. Talk to someone. Take a walk. Do a crossword puzzle. Finish the laundry. Drive somewhere. Turn on the television. Listen to music. Meditate. Focus on your senses. What are you feeling, seeing, smelling, or hearing? Almost any distraction will do. Make a list of noneating activities you find engaging and nurturing so that when a craving strikes, you're ready for it.
3. Don't give your attention to ego-based thoughts (especially negative ones), thoughts that are about "me" or "my story" or that start with "I," such as "I like, I want, I don't want, I hope, I don't like, I feel, I think, I believe, I can't, I won't, I'm not, I did..." This involvement with the "me" is what gave you the craving crazies in the first place.

Powerful Kung Fu #10: Get Engaged in What You're Doing

1. Notice that a craving is on the scene and get yourself the heck out of the kitchen!
2. Become engaged and focus completely on whatever you're doing now, whether it's work, running an errand, vacuuming, finishing a good book, or making a call. When you're really absorbed in something, you can go for hours without a single thought about food.

Powerful Kung Fu #11: Pick a "9" or "10"

1. Notice that a craving is on the scene and get yourself the heck out of the kitchen!
2. Pick a "9" or "10" from your Pleasure Scale list. Take a break from whatever was causing your hand to reach for food and do something you love instead.

Powerful Kung Fu #12: I Do That, Too

1. Notice that a craving is on the scene and get yourself the heck out of the kitchen!
2. If you're angry or feel hurt because someone did something you didn't like, remember a time that you did or said the same sort of thing and forgive that person. It's hard to stay angry at someone when we find the same failing in ourselves. To keep yourself from stuffing the feeling with food and heal instead, see your own failing, and forgive yourself and the other person.

Powerful Kung Fu #13: Dis-identify with the Stressful Thought

1. Notice that a craving is on the scene and get yourself the heck out of the kitchen!
2. Ask yourself, **"What stressful thought am I believing right now?"** or **"What story am I in?"** Wait for the answer.
3. When the answer comes, ask yourself, **"What is noticing this belief?"** This is a powerful question because it helps you dis-identify with the thought.
4. Say to yourself, **"Oh, thank goodness, it's just a stressful belief—it's not me. It couldn't be me because I'm over here, noticing it."**

Powerful Kung Fu #14: Inquire

1. Notice that a craving is on the scene and get yourself the heck out of the kitchen!

2. Notice that you're upset and address the upset directly using inquiry. Do this by asking yourself, **"What story am I telling myself that's causing me to feel this way right now? What am I believing?"**

3. When you discover the belief, take it to inquiry by asking the following questions:

    o **Can I know beyond a shadow of a doubt that this belief is true?** Even if you believe that it's true, go on to the next question.

    o **What is the opposite of this belief? Could that be as true or truer?** Come up with evidence to support the opposite belief. If the opposite of the belief is also true, perhaps the original negative belief isn't true after all! This discovery helps you to stop believing the stressful thought.

Powerful Kung Fu #15: Think Something Positive Instead

1. Notice that a craving is on the scene and get yourself the heck out of the kitchen!

2. Replace the negative thought that's generating the feeling with a positive one. For example, replace **"Nothing's going right today"** with **"Everything's going right today."** Then come up with evidence to support the positive thought. This kung fu can be a bit of a slippery slope because it does keep you in the realm of thought, and when you're in thought, it's easy to go back to spinning a negative story and feeding the feeling again.

Powerful Kung Fu #16: Not Now—Maybe Later

1. Notice that a craving is on the scene and get yourself the heck out of the kitchen!
2. Recognize that the Child is on the scene and talk to her the way you would talk to a child who is pestering you about getting something that you don't want to give her right now. Tell her, **"Not now—maybe later."**

Powerful Kung Fu #17: Just This Once…

1. Notice that a craving is on the scene and get yourself the heck out of the kitchen!
2. Rather than treading the well-worn path of self-soothing through food, try something different just this once. Don't give in to the usual urge—for now. You can always decide to do that later, if that's what you want, but for now, move out of the kitchen.

Powerful Kung Fu #18: Am I Hungry? (The Cottage Cheese Test)

1. Notice that a craving is on the scene and get yourself the heck out of the kitchen!
2. Ask yourself if you are physically hungry. This is different from just wanting to taste something nice. One of my workshop participants uses what she calls "the cottage cheese test." She likes cottage cheese, but the only time she actually wants to eat it is when she's truly hungry. If she could eat cottage cheese, she knows she's hungry. If she couldn't eat cottage cheese and she wants to eat something, she knows that she's not physically hungry and something else is going on. If you answer no when you ask yourself if you're physically hungry, ask yourself, **"What's going on that's causing me to want to move toward food when I'm not hungry?"**

My Process

After many, many months, I learned to see the whole truth about food in the moment I felt the impulse to reach for it. I began by setting the intention to bring more awareness to my pattern. Because I had years and years of compulsive eating under my belt (literally!), it took a while to change it.

Here's the whole truth of overeating pleasure food: It comes out to 5% "taste good" (for the few short minutes that it spends in your mouth) and 95% bloat, weight gain, ill health, guilt, shame, blame, self-deprecation, and perpetual low self-esteem. Once I really saw this, I could no longer pretend that I hadn't seen it. Once you stop believing in Santa Claus, you can't just decide to believe in him again. The jig is up.

It's the same with seeing the whole truth about food. It took many, many repetitions of seeing the whole truth of overeating in the midst of a compulsive impulse for me to finally be able to interrupt it. Most of the time, I would catch it after the fact. At first, I'd remember the whole truth about food after an episode. Then, after some practice, I was able to see it during the episode and interrupt it. Finally, I was able to notice the uncomfortable feeling at the same time I felt the impulse to reach for food. At that point, I was able to see the whole truth about food, and choose not to follow the impulse.

Here's the skinny on my healing process:

Phase One: Noticing after the fact. At first it seemed impossible to interrupt my automatic eating response. Instead, my noticing tended to come in *after* my emotional eating. After some initial feelings of disappointment that I hadn't been able to catch it sooner, I would do a postmortem and imagine what it would have been like if I'd been able to use one of the emotional-eating kung fu exercises. My work in Phase One was learning to be gentle with myself and forgive myself for not being able to break this habit perfectly.

Phase Two: Noticing during an emotional-eating attack. Next, I noticed that I was eating emotionally *while* I was doing it and chose to stop by using one of the emotional-eating kung fus. I was able to stop sooner and sooner. At first, choice came in after I'd been eating unconsciously for about five minutes, then three minutes, then two, and so on.

Phase Three: Noticing before an emotional-eating attack is about to happen. In time, I was able to notice the impulse to eat emotionally and catch it *before* I acted on it. I was able to use one of the kung fus to notice the feeling, thought, or need and deal with it directly rather than stuffing it with food. Phase Three can be a long time in coming—perhaps years—and even after it shows up, you can still move back to Phase Two or even Phase One intermittently. Sticking with it, however, can lead to freedom.

Chapter Summary

- ❏ Remember to see the whole truth about food rather than the Child's sliver of truth about it.
- ❏ Remember all of the unpleasant consequences of overeating a pleasure food:
  - ○ Feeling guilty about eating unhealthily and not being strong enough to stop
  - ○ Ill health
  - ○ Not fitting into clothes
  - ○ Wanting to hide because you feel too fat
  - ○ Weight gain
  - ○ Low self-esteem
  - ○ Losing confidence professionally and socially
  - ○ Feeling bloated, nauseated, or listless
- ❏ The Child gets activated when we experience a craving and says, "I have to have this right now!"

❑ When we're identified with the Child and we get a craving, it feels like a life or death imperative.

❑ You weaken the Child when you decide not to respond to her every time she shows up.

❑ If you're willing to see that an irrational part of yourself has been running the show, then you can begin to develop a more rational approach to eating.

❑ Eating is so quick—so fleeting.

❑ Seeing that the pleasure you get from eating is fleeting is liberating. It helps you realize that not having two minutes with a particular food won't impact your life.

❑ If eating is the best thing ever, why do we need to pair it with other activities?

❑ Remember to use the list of powerful kung fus for cravings and emotional eating that starts on page 50.

❑ How you think about food is what makes it seem so wonderful, desirable, meaningful, and important.

❑ When you see how untrue and overblown your thinking is about food, you're on your way to thinking differently and healing your relationship with food.

To-Do List

Check off any task that you have fully or partially completed:

❑ I'm becoming more aware of my food thoughts.

❑ I'm learning to distinguish between the problematic thoughts that come from the Child and the pragmatic thoughts that come from the Wise Witness.

❑ I successfully ignored a thought from the Child.

❑ I spent time feeding my soul.

❑ I made a plan to spend time feeding my soul each day.

❑ I was able to see the whole picture of food rather than getting hooked by the Child's promise of taste pleasure.

❑ I used the following powerful kung fus for cravings and emotional eating:

_____

_____

_____

❑ I discovered which kung fu for cravings and emotional eating works best for me.

❑ I tried using a kung fu for cravings and emotional eating, even if it was after a bout of emotional eating.

❑ I've been gentle and patient with myself when I've indulged a craving or engaged in emotional eating.

❑ Even if I haven't been able to be tender with myself, I noticed that tendency to be harsh, set the intention to be kinder to myself next time, and forgave myself.

❑ I made a list of my "9's" and "10's."

CHAPTER 3

The Second Step: Wise Food Choices

•◆•

Congratulations! You made it through the First Step and are hopefully bringing more awareness to your food thoughts and changing your relationship with food!

On to the Second Step, Wise Food Choices. Making wise food choices means getting most of your calories from healthy, nutritious, whole foods like fruit, vegetables, seeds, nuts, grains, and meats—eventually. What do I mean by eventually? This is your life and your process. Because everyone is different, you'll be making changes on *your* timetable, going at the pace that feels right for you. For some people, that means cutting out most junk food cold turkey right now. For others, it means limiting Twinkies six months from now. But the sooner you start implementing the Second Step, the easier and happier your life will be.

Making wise food choices means eating with health in mind—eating foods that make sense for the optimal functioning of your body. It's common sense. Every day, you'll want to make sure you get protein, carbohydrates, and healthy fats from whole, unprocessed foods. Ideally, each meal would be balanced in this way, too.

You don't need to be rigid about this, so please don't turn this step into another stick to beat yourself up with. The body is adaptable, and it's okay to eat for pleasure sometimes as long as *eventually* most of your calories are nutritious calories. If you're not sure how to eat healthily, read a good book on nutrition (see the Recommended Reading section at the end of this book) or visit a nutritionist.

Here's how to start putting the Second Step into practice: When you're hungry, rather than imagining what would taste good right now, go to your rational mind and ask, "What could my body use right now?" If you haven't been eating or thinking about food this way, it's not surprising. Our culture doesn't support this way of thinking about food. It tends to encourage the Child's romanticization of food.

As you read this chapter, if negative thoughts come up, like "Good God, if I eat this way, I'll be miserable. Eating won't be any fun. My pleasure in life comes from food. It's the only thing I have, and now I have to give that up, too!" jot them down. At the end of this chapter, we'll take these thoughts to inquiry, a handy tool for debunking and rendering impotent any negative or stressful thoughts.

You *can* do this!! If I can get free after a 35-year eating obsession, anyone can. Good luck and have fun!

Meshuga!

If my Grandpa Sam could see the way we eat these days, he'd say that it was meshuga! (That's Yiddish for *crazy*.) We are cramming junk into our mouths and eating *it* instead of food. How nuts is that? We like how junk tastes, but once it leaves our mouths, there's nothing our bodies can do with it. If our cells could talk, they'd ask, "What the heck are you doing up there? When are you going to give me something I can use?" In our culture, judging from our expanding bodies, we seem to think that food is anything that tastes good that we can cram down our gullets.

Imagine aliens landing on Earth from a more advanced civilization and seeing us converting perfectly good, whole food into nonfood, and then stuffing ourselves with it until our bellies hurt. The aliens would watch in amazement as we process wheat kernels by removing so much of their nutritional value that we have to enrich the flour afterwards. What could motivate this strange behavior? "Somewhere along the way," they'd surmise, "Earthlings must have decided that white is the best food color and smooth and fluffy are the best textures." My guess is that the aliens would think we were a few beans short of a burrito, and with good reason.

Strangely, we treat our pets and cars better than our bodies. At least we feed them what they eat. We feed dogs dog food, not parakeet or cat food. When cars are thirsty, we fill them with diesel or gasoline because that's what they drink. If one day our mechanic suggested that we fuel our car with orange juice, we'd think he'd lost it and take our business elsewhere. Everyone knows cars don't drink orange juice!

Yet when it comes to our bodies, we're like the misguided mechanic. We know deep down that our bodies run on whole food, but we continue to feed them junk. We seek the taste pleasure of nonfoods like candy, cookies, donuts, and potato chips and at the same time we want to strut around in sexy, thin bodies. The problem is that bodies that eat junk get fat, sluggish, moody, and sick, just as cars that are filled with the wrong fuel don't run well or seize up. It's a simple law of mechanics.

Food Is Grown, Junk Is Made

Junk food pairs two unrelated terms: junk—sugary or salty processed stuff with little or no nutritional value (nonfood)—and food. Food is grown or raised and contains nutrients that the body needs. Junk is made. It's processed and refined, designed primarily to tantalize our palates. This is an important distinction to keep in mind as you take the Second Step.

Food, Sex, and Skinny Thinking

The obvious question is: "Why are we eating stuff that's not food?" Well, because it tastes so darn good. We're hooked on the pleasure of eating rich, sweet, and salty foods that look, smell, and taste divine and delight all of our senses. The food industry creates products with this in mind. We consume these products, which alter our metabolism and train our taste buds to desire them, and the food industry further fuels demand for them through alluring advertising. This is a brilliant marketing coup for corporations and an insidious exchange for us—the food companies get fat bottom lines, and we just get fat bottoms!

Here are some examples of pleasure food advertising:

"Do you dream in chocolate?"
"Once you break its shell, the filling will start to melt and so will you."
"Over 160 years of passion for that one moment of yours."

These taglines come to us courtesy of Lindt, and they're good examples of how food marketers do their best to entice us to lust after their products. Selling food based on nutrition isn't sexy, so their tactics appeal to our desire for pleasure, working us into a craving frenzy so that we feel compelled to race out in hot pursuit of their products. If we're not flushed with desire after seeing an ad, it hasn't done its job.

Sometimes, it's the consumers themselves who feed these fantasies. Here is what one of Lindt's customers wrote:

"Lindt Lindor Truffles are the ultimate chocolate lover's dream. The wonderful smooth chocolate filling inside a rich chocolate shell is enough to turn a chocolate lover into a truffle addict. I bought a couple bags of the milk and white chocolate as favors for a party and just couldn't seem to control my urge to eat them all. Just one of them will get you hooked."

Having learned the potent trick of selling the sizzle, not the steak, food marketers' first line of attack is our senses. If they succeed in engaging our senses through a seductive image, they lead us down the merry path of imagining just how good that food will taste once it's in our mouth. At that point, they've got us. Just by encouraging us to imagine what their food will taste like, they make us their food slaves.

Marketers have been co-opted by the ego, which makes them the mouthpiece of the Child. Her main job when it comes to food is getting us to eat entertaining food, enticing us based on the imagined taste pleasure food will deliver. The problem with letting your eating be guided by food marketing or the Child is that it's like believing the "happily ever after" line in a movie or fairy tale—you never get to see what happens after the movie ends, so you don't know how things turn out. The guy gets the girl and then what?

It's the same way with eating pleasure food. You experience the intense pleasure hit while the food is in your mouth, but then what? To keep that sensation going, you need to take another bite and then another, and so on. At some point, those bites don't taste very good, and your stomach protests. The pleasure turns into pain. The attraction turns into repulsion. As your body struggles to digest the junk, you feel bloated, headachy, groggy, and grumpy. Your body suffers because not only did it not receive the nutrients it needs, it now has to expend precious energy to get rid of the junk. To top it off, it may have to carry around excess weight as a result of this pleasure food party.

The bottom line is this: If you want to avoid the pull of the Child and negate her influence on your eating life, avoid sexy food ads. Turn away from any images or sound bites that quicken your pulse and get you salivating. When the Child encourages you to imagine what food tastes like, ignore those thoughts. If you follow them, you may find yourself careening down a slippery slope and landing smack-dab in the middle of an over-the-top pleasure food party.

Food versus Entertainment

Generally, the pleasure foods that you can't stop eating have—surprise, surprise—almost no nutrition. You couldn't survive on them. As a culture, we've fooled ourselves into thinking that pleasure food is food, but it's not. It's entertainment. Don't delude yourself into thinking that the junk you're ingesting is food. If you do, you're going to replace real food with entertaining junk and think you're getting the nutrition you need. You might be getting a tiny bit of nutrition from it, but even that comes at a very high cost.

If you see pleasure food as entertainment, you'll be less likely to replace good food with it, and it will hold a smaller place in your life. Just like you don't watch television all day long or go to the movies every night because you have other things to do, it's unhealthy to eat pleasure food too often. You watch a television show at night or go to a movie once a week. Similarly, maybe you have a little pleasure food at night or make a conscious decision to entertain yourself with it one night a week.

Eating Processed Fast Food Means Choosing Taste over Health

For the most part, fast-food restaurants are eating minefields. There are a few notable exceptions, such as Whole Foods Market, SUBWAY, Panera Bread, and UFood Grill, that offer fresh, whole food options and provide nutritional information. Most other fast-food chains cater to pleasure through taste, choosing to make their offerings taste a certain way at the expense of nutrition so their foods can compete in the marketplace. What do they do to make food taste good? They add fat, salt, and sugar.

Most restaurants use considerably more fat, salt, and sugar than we would at home. A restaurant's motive is profit, not our health, and creating food that tastes better than the competition's is the key to filling its coffers. If we're to bring our bodies back into balance, though, we need to ask ourselves, "Is taste more important than health?"

We've been focused on taste from the time we were children, and our taste buds have become accustomed to the flavors of pleasure foods, expecting them every time we eat. But now that we're adults, it's time to take responsibility for our eating and tell ourselves the truth: Most food companies and restaurants sell unhealthy foods that human bodies were never designed to eat, and if we want to get healthy and stay at a natural weight, we have to stop or limit our junk eating.

If you're overweight, you're probably eating a lot of fat and sugar, perhaps more than you even know, which dramatically throws off your metabolism and your relationship to food. It's difficult to comprehend the full impact of this way of eating because you're accustomed to it and, to a certain extent, your body has adapted to it. To reverse this unnatural trend, you've got to eliminate most of the junk in favor of fresh, whole, unprocessed foods.

You don't need to become rigid or completely pure in your eating, though. The body is adaptable and can handle most foods if you don't inundate it with processed stuff. Giving it the appropriate amount of produce and whole, natural foods reacclimates your taste buds to the food you were designed to eat. Once that happens, eating healthily becomes easy and—believe it or not—preferable! Why? Because you end up enjoying nutritious foods more than you ever enjoyed the junk. Also, when you reduce the amount of fat, salt, and sugar you're consuming, the difference in your energy level and feeling of well-being is dramatic.

Pleasure Food

For food lovers, eating almost any food is pretty darn pleasurable, so "pleasure food" is at best redundant. But let's dig deeper. Pleasure food is any tantalizing edible that sets your heart atwitter. It's the stuff you fantasize about, longingly counting the minutes before getting it into your mouth.

As I said earlier, pleasure food has been engineered, often through the addition of fat, salt, and sugar, to captivate us and get us to crave it. Food executives have sized us up, found our Achilles' heels, and designed products so delicious we can't resist them. Even when we're eating them, all we can think about is being able to eat more. The proof is in the pudding. Witness the fact that we can never get enough potato chips, ice cream, or chocolate chip cookies to satisfy us, so most of us keep eating them long after our bellies are aching.

The trickiest part of the whole scheme is that not only do food companies make food that we can't stop eating, *they have remade us.* Eating their addictive products rewired our taste buds and metabolisms. The companies created the products and now those same products have re-created us to be their perfect consumers.

"Okay," you might say, "I can see how feeling out of control around pleasure food and eating too much of it is not a good thing. We've all been lured into a trap and now we're suffering from the resulting overweight and ill health. But what's the alternative? Boring food? Who the heck wants to eat that?" Hold on for a minute and hear me out.

Food, which was once nice-tasting fuel for the body, has become a much bigger deal. It has become a celebrity, a superstar, a guilty pleasure of biblical proportions. The questions you have to ask yourself are: Do I want food to loom so large in my life? Do I want it to dominate my waking consciousness? Is there more to life than lusting after, craving, and avoiding food? If somewhere deep down in the recesses of your consciousness, you know that living this way is not really living, but indentured servitude, it's time to get your power back.

For me, freedom has meant not eating much pleasure food. I cut most of it out and my taste buds quickly readjusted to their natural state. As a result, healthy food, food that's grown, not made, tastes every bit as good as pleasure food used to. In other words, I haven't given up anything!

My so-called boring food tastes anything but boring to me. Most of my diet is made up of fresh fruits, vegetables, protein, nuts, nut butters, seeds, brown rice, and oats. That diet may not get your heart racing, but I'm perfectly satisfied eating this way. Although I occasionally eat some borderline foods, like baked tortilla chips and popcorn, I've lost my desire for the junk.

A while ago, I decided to bake a treat. Using bananas for a sweetener, oat flour, and very little butter, I made apple pecan bread. Even though I didn't classify it as junk, the bread tasted so good, so exciting, that I ate way more than I had intended. I felt out of control and disappointed in myself.

Through this experience, I learned how important freedom is to me. It's more important than a fleeting good taste in my mouth. Now if I eat something that makes me feel out of control, I don't make it or bring it into my house again. To most people, my food is boring. But I'll take boring any day. It tastes better than the junk ever did, it's truly nutritious and satisfying, keeps me effortlessly healthy and slim, and doesn't leave me wanting more. And that's pretty darn exciting!

Look What She Can Eat!

In my workshops, I can always count on hearing some version of the following complaint at least once: "I see these darn skinny people. There they are at the table across from me, shoveling in French fries with both hands. How can this be if there is a just God? Here I am giving up bread and measuring out my chopped celery just so I can walk without causing an earthquake, and they get to eat whatever their skinny little hearts desire. It's not fair!"

We assume that others get to have it both ways. That they get to eat their fill of pleasure food and still fit into their size-two skinny jeans. But we really don't know what their story is. Maybe they *are* the rare specimens who can eat whatever they want and not gain an ounce. Chances are, though, that something else is going on.

When we spy a skinny junk-food eater doing her thing, it could be that we've just caught her in the midst of a "double whammy." That's when you skip real food to save calories and move straight to the junk. The term viscerally describes the wallop it gives to the body. Skipping real food in favor of junk means depriving the body of important nutrition (whammy #1). The body then has to expend energy to get rid of the junk that's been dumped into it (whammy #2).

The skinny junk-food eater might not gain weight, but her body pays for this practice with diminished energy levels or a compromised immune system. The double whammy is a dangerous strategy for balancing the two mutually exclusive egoic desires of wanting to look good and wanting to eat our favorite pleasure foods. Even skinny junk-food eaters can only fool the body for so long. Sooner or later, everybody pays the price.

In the end, the only real payoff anybody gets from the "look what she can eat" lament is being able to add another chapter to their woe-is-me story. "Woe is me because she has something that I don't. Look at how God left me off her Christmas list…again!" But anytime we compare ourselves with others and come up short, we can be sure that we are identified with the ego.

From egoic consciousness, we presume to understand the wisdom of life's plan for us and find fault with it. We assume that we're not getting our due and others are. In those moments, we forget who we are. In presuming that we are mere mortals whose happiness rests on pleasure seeking and desire fulfillment, we have no idea how short we sell ourselves. We cut ourselves off from our true selves and miss seeing the innumerable ways that we have been blessed. We mistake the challenges that serve our evolution for being forsaken by God, when, in fact, within the challenges lie the seeds of our awakening. To envy another's path is to deny grace and miss the bounty that is naturally ours in every moment.

It Feels Better to Feel Better Longer

A friend of mine shared that he used to love to eat sugary cookies. One day, he said, he was looking at a plate of cookies, imagining how heavenly they would taste. Then he stopped and remembered his past experiences with them. He thought back to how awful he felt after eating them, not just once, but every time. With this in mind, he decided to pass on the cookies, concluding, "It feels better to feel better longer."

My friend was able to say no to the Child tempting him by seeing the whole truth of the experience. By choosing to forgo the intense but short-lived taste pleasure from eating the cookies, he was able to avoid the longer period of physical discomfort that would inevitably follow. Seeing the whole picture of eating the cookies removed the compelling desire for them.

The Child plays the same game with us over and over again until we get wise to it. She hooks us with a small sliver of truth—pleasure food tastes good—and leaves out the rest of the truth. Now don't get me wrong. There is a place for eating entertaining food. But if we want to maintain healthy, slim bodies without worry or struggle, then that place is a small place. To feel better longer, we need to get the bulk of our calories from healthy, whole foods like fruits, vegetables, and whole grains, not from pleasure foods.

Why Wait for Health Issues?

Health scares can be so traumatic that we do an about-face in our eating. Oddly enough, when this happens, good fortune is smiling on us. Nothing helps us prioritize health faster than the prospect of the grim reaper knocking at our door. But do we really need to wait for a crisis? Why not embrace the possibility of choosing health over taste now? Doesn't waking up to the truth of how we're feeding our bodies *before* a health scare strikes make a lot more sense?

My Name Is Laura, and I'm a Sugarholic…

At a fancy restaurant one evening when I was 10, my family and I settled into our table, and a glittering array of sugar cubes in an ornate silver bowl caught my eye. Quietly, I lifted one with the tiny spoon and hid it behind my roll. When no one was looking, I ate it, then moved on to another cube, chain-eating them as if they were the main course.

When my parents heard my crunching, they implored me to stop my embarrassing, uncouth behavior. So, my sister and I came up with a new plan—secretly lining our socks with the precious cubes. When it was time to leave, we walked out in full view of the other patrons, our socks bulging with sugar cubes. Our unsuspecting parents were horrified. So begins the tale of my sugar addiction.

Refined white sugar is a pleasure drug. If you don't believe me, just put a spoonful on your tongue and observe the instantaneous effects. You'll experience a warming, comfortable sensation that makes you feel safe and happy. Sugary foods aren't called comfort foods by accident.

Until recently, I assumed that I was a foodaholic, addicted to the food I liked, but now I've learned that my compulsive overeating had two parts: 1) responding to uncomfortable emotions by stuffing food and 2) responding to physical cravings arising from my sugar and chocolate addictions.

I came from a nice family, attended college, and had a career and family of my own. I never thought of myself as an addict, except in a jocular sort of way. To do so would have meant seeing myself differently—not as a nice, respectable, successful girl, but as a drug addict who needed her fix.

And that would have been too hard to swallow. After all, I wasn't breaking into people's homes in search of a Toblerone bar or a homemade chocolate chip cookie. Yet when a craving struck, it was hard to think about anything else. I finally had to admit that I was indeed a sugar junkie.

Now that I think about it, quesadillas and pizza slices were never the main attractions of a binge for me. I love those foods, and I might have misjudged and accidentally overeaten them, but I never binged just on them. There was always a saturation point. Those savory foods were the small towns I traveled through en route to my big city destination—sugar.

To see if you've formed an addictive relationship with sugar, you only need to ask one question: Do I crave it? If the answer is yes, then at some point in your life, probably when you were a child, you became a sugar junkie. There's no shame in this. Adults constantly give kids sugary food, and candy and sugary cereals are marketed almost exclusively to children. However, when we consistently feed kids addictive drugs, we can hardly be surprised when they get hooked.

Thinking you can be moderate if you've become a sugar addict is self-delusion. You quip, "Of course I can be moderate. I only ate one biscotti last night, so how can I be an addict?" I asked the same thing. I'll tell you one thing, though, there was never a time when there was no sugar in my house. And my grocery carts always managed to position themselves smack-dab in the middle of the sweets aisle. Sure, I could be moderate. Sometimes I could even go for months without overdoing it. But then something would happen, a negative emotion would rear its ugly head, and I would binge. Unfortunately, it wasn't just sugar I was addicted to.

...I'm Also a Chocoholic

Chocolate has been my sacred love and passion for as long as I can remember. My favorite kind as a child was Bavarian chocolates. Once in a blue moon, the luscious, dark chocolate-mint squares would make a cameo appearance at our house.

One day, we were having company, and for some reason I found myself alone in the rear of the house. To my delight and surprise, I found a virgin box of Bavarian chocolates! I couldn't believe my luck—a whole box all to myself. My exultation was unsullied by any urge to share. No, by gosh, I found them, and finders keepers! I wasn't sharing them with anyone.

One after the other, I crammed them into my mouth, barely giving myself time to chew one before loading in another. I must have gotten at least halfway through the box when I felt it—a powerful contraction in my stomach followed by a wave of nausea.

Thankfully, the bathroom was close by, because the chocolates came back up even more quickly than they'd gone down. I'd always thought I had a cast-iron constitution, but my digestive tract was no match for my capacity to chain-eat chocolates.

I used to call myself a chocoholic, like it was an adorable quirk that endeared me to others. So many of my friends shared this chocolate fetish that it was like we were all members of a secret society. Instead of gathering in dark alleys, though, we gathered at darkened corner tables in out-of-the-way bakery cafes. And instead of a secret handshake, we shared chocolate confections that sent us into states of ecstasy.

Finding another chocolate lover was like finding a fellow worshipper in the same offbeat religion. You could let your hair down and admit that you, too, were a worshipper of Nestlé, Godiva, Fanny May, or Lindt. Instantly, you knew this was someone you could hang out with who wouldn't shame or judge you. In the realm of addictions, being a chocoholic was innocuous—no worse than collecting shoes or watching soap operas—or so we rationalized. It certainly didn't carry the stigma of alcoholism or drug addiction.

Being a chocoholic is so common that it's actually a feather in our cap. It humanizes us. When people know we love chocolate, they can say, "Oh, so-and-so is just like us. She has a weakness." Not only does being a chocoholic carry no stigma, it's socially acceptable—after all, we're very easy to shop for! Abstaining, on the other hand, makes us an object of curiosity and causes others to fidget in their chairs. Like it or not, our abstinence makes them consider this possibility for themselves, and often, they don't want to go there.

Why Listening to the Body Doesn't Work

For most of my adult life, I've been trying to cure my eating issues by putting my body back in charge, figuring that it possessed an innate wisdom that I was clearly lacking. My two eating guidelines were:

1. Eat only when hungry and stop when full.
2. Imagine what my body wants to eat. Is it something cold or hot, sweet or savory, etc.?

Yet when I tried to put the second guideline into practice, I kept running into the same snag. Too often, when I tuned into what my body wanted, it would say, "Something chocolate, please." Even though I had only a rudimentary knowledge of nutrition, something told me that chocolate for breakfast, lunch, and dinner couldn't be healthy. So what was going on? Was my body defective? Was there a short circuit in its signaling system?

Of course, when I did follow the second guideline and indulge my body's chocolate craving, following the first guideline—stopping when I was full—became nearly impossible. Consequently, my pattern became: 1) listen to what my body wants, 2) gain weight, 3) diet to get it off, and 4) try to develop a healthy relationship with food by going back to the seemingly sensible approach of letting body wisdom guide my eating.

What I didn't understand at the time was that my body was physically addicted to sugar and chocolate, and as a result, when I asked it what it wanted, it most often answered, "Something sweet or chocolaty." After many years, I concluded that letting my body guide my eating didn't work. There was no freedom in letting my body continue to eat foods that left me feeling powerless and out of control.

Listening to our bodies to decide how to eat doesn't work these days because we're eating the wrong foods. The messages from a body that's addicted to junk are simply not a reliable guide to healthy eating. Pleasure food was created to entice us to eat it and throw off our taste buds and our body's signals for hunger and satiation.

The truth is, as nice as the idea sounds, we really can't talk to our bodies. Although our bodies have some unconscious input into our eating—like when my girlfriend was anemic during her pregnancy and dreamt of liver sausage—we can't pick up the phone and dial our bodies to ask for guidance about what to eat. We can't communicate with our bodies on a conscious level.

If you want to know what to eat, the best strategy is to eat primarily foods that are grown rather than made and to educate yourself about portion size. When it's time to eat, use the wise adult part of yourself, the Wise Witness, to help you create a balanced meal. To begin to get your power back and establish a healthy, rational relationship with food, stop listening to your body and work to heal your food addictions.

Here is a list of many of the pleasure foods that can keep you struggling with your health and weight:

List of Pleasure Foods

Physically & Emotionally Addictive	Emotionally Addictive
Foods made with sugar and/or chocolate:	Salty fried foods:
Bakery goods	*Potato chips, French fries*
Ice cream	Salty foods:
Candy	*Pretzels, popcorn*
Chocolates	Starchy foods:
Soft drinks	*Pancakes, waffles, bread*
Milkshakes	Salty fatty foods:
	Butter, cheese, nuts, hot dogs
	Fatty starchy foods:
	Pizza, quesadillas

When you have an emotional relationship with a food, you crave it and feel giddy and excited around it. You may feel a frenzied compulsion to eat it not five minutes from now, but right now! You look forward to eating it and often eat past satiety because you enjoy the taste. You turn to it when you're looking for comfort, a treat, or an escape from uncomfortable feelings. Rarely able to eat just one bite, you feel impotent and weak-willed around it. Stressful thoughts about your relationship to this food undermine your self-esteem and cause even more destruction by triggering your conditioned pattern of eating it when you're upset.

Although you probably already have a good idea about which foods make you feel out of control, it's helpful to clearly identify them. Use the following questions to see if you're on the right track. Start by filling in the blanks with "celery":

1. Does the prospect of eating _____ make you giddy and excited?
2. Do you have a hard time limiting how much _____ you eat? Can you easily eat just one bite and stop?
3. Does eating _____ or having it around make you feel powerless and out of control?

Did you answer yes to any of the questions? That's hard to imagine. People generally don't get addicted to celery, carrots, or Brussels sprouts; they get addicted to junk. Use the three questions to start compiling your list of addictive foods. Choose a favorite food and if you can answer yes to any of the questions, add it to your list.

A Grown-up Relationship with Food

When you were a child, what foods did you comfort yourself with? What did you eat to distract yourself when you were in pain? Most of us developed an emotional relationship with sugar when we were children because adults gave us sweets as rewards and treats, to show us they were feeling good about us. As a result, we associated sweet things with positive feelings, love, and approval. So when we're looking to reward ourselves for a job well done or console ourselves if we're upset or when we just want to do something nice for ourselves, many of us have long turned to sugar. Given the physical addictiveness of sugar and the powerful emotional associations we have with it, it's no wonder we have trouble controlling ourselves around it!

Understanding that your underlying beliefs about food generate a certain relationship with it helps you step back and begin to choose whether you'll indulge in pleasure food as a reward or not and whether you'll continue that relationship pattern. Seeing your relationship with food as a conditioned one that you formed as a child can help you begin to develop the more rational, adult part of you. You can say to yourself, "Oh yes, I can see that I've been conditioned to see that as a reward, but you know what? I've had enough rewards today, and I don't need to keep going in that direction. That's not good for my body."

Conditioning creates an overblown relationship with food, causing us to see it as our lover, our friend, and our source of fulfillment. As a result, we think we need it to be happy. But we don't. Once you begin to see that, you can choose to change your relationship by questioning your beliefs. Acknowledging that your conditioning is causing you to sacrifice your health and emotional well-being means you can no longer be fooled by it. You step outside of it and move beyond it rather than continuing to react to it. From that place, there is freedom. There is choice.

Where's the Parent?

Thinking of food as a reward is only a problem if you reward yourself too much. When there's no parent there to say, "Hey, honey, you've had enough cookies," the Child says, "Whoopee! There's nobody here to stop me, so I can have as many cookies as I want." But every Child needs a parent.

Just because you're grown and there isn't an adult telling you when to stop doesn't mean you can eat whatever you want and not pay a price. If you want to permanently solve your weight and food issues, you need to develop the adult inside of you, or that Child's just going to keep chasing after the treats.

Most of us experience having a more mature relationship with food when we're on a diet. At those times, the diet book becomes the parent. But unless you integrate that parent, you'll go back to your old ways as soon as the diet's over. You have to build a relationship with your own inner parent, your Wise Witness.

Your Wise Witness is an aspect of yourself that has always been there, but you may not have noticed it because you were so busy listening to the Child. It's that objective place within you that is able to choose to follow your conditioning or not. The more often you align with the Wise Witness, the easier it becomes. The spiritual aspect of healing your food issues includes developing the sense of yourself as this Wise Witness who sees the whole picture, isn't buffeted by conditioning, and can choose whether to indulge or not.

Taking Back Our Power over Food

Why would we do something as irrational as eating food that has no nutritional value? Because it tastes good. We crave the taste, and how do we stop wanting what we want? The simple answer is that we can't. We can't push against desire because we're always too late.

The only way to stop *wanting* a food is to decide that it's no longer in your life. Then you stop thinking about it and, if you're not thinking about it, you can't desire it. Here's how this works: Imagine that you're walking by a bakery with a friend. She wants a cookie and asks if you want one, too. You respond, "You go ahead. I don't eat cookies anymore."

For most of us, a namby-pamby stance like "I'll cut down first" or "I'll give it up for Lent" just won't work. If you know you're going back to it, you'll be thinking about it, lighting candles for it, and holding all-night vigils awaiting its return.

The small percentage of people who can exercise power over the foods they're addicted to without abstaining completely have found a strategy that works for them. Maybe they eat addictive foods only when they're out, or set rules that limit the quantities and times they allow themselves to eat the stuff. For example, "I won't keep this in the house, but I can eat it when I'm at a restaurant"; "I can have this once a week when I go to Aunt Sallie's for dinner"; or "I will eat a small square of this and *only that much* and freeze the rest." For the majority of us, though, these strategies can be very hard to stick to.

We like to tell ourselves that we can eat pleasure food in moderation. We're not wimps, after all. Just look at all the successful diets we've been on! We're grown-ups, and we can control ourselves around these foods that have become the main way we treat ourselves and get pleasure in life. And that's true—except when it isn't, when we lose it and overeat in response to a physical or emotional craving. We need to get real about this if we want a sane relationship with food. If we are ever to overcome our addiction, we need to face the music and take back our power over food.

If you feel out of control over a certain food, either limit it using a strategy that works for you, or cut it out of your life.

How Do I Stop Wanting What I Want?

The secret to being able to stop eating pleasure food is to *stop wanting it*. Well, duh! Forgive me for stating the obvious. It's reasonable to posit that if you didn't *want* to eat pleasure food, you couldn't overeat, and you couldn't get fat. But how do you stop wanting pleasure food, particularly when you are in the habit of eating it?

When I was in the brownie business, people often asked me if being around brownies all day made me immune to their charms. I wish! The more I ate brownies, the more I wanted them. In fact, *the more you eat any pleasure food, the more you want it*, and the more you want it, the more you eat it. It's a vicious circle.

The idea of giving up a food we love is tantamount to giving up our right arm or our firstborn child. Even King Solomon wouldn't be able to come up with a solution to the problem of passionately loving food that doesn't love us back. So what to do? Although it seems counterintuitive, *the only way to stop wanting a food is to stop eating it*. Here's why:

⚘ When you stop eating the food and decide that it's out of your life forever—not just for a day or a week or a month—you stop thinking about it.
⚘ When you stop thinking about it, you stop desiring it.

We're used to thinking, "Gosh, if I stop eating this food that I love, I'll feel deprived and want it all the more." This is true if you cut out pleasure foods temporarily, but *if you decide that those foods are no longer in your life, you stop thinking about them*. And if you stop thinking about them, you stop craving them. If you stop craving them, you stop eating them, and—wonder of wonders—you lose weight! It takes thought to create desire. No thought, no desire. It's just that simple.

No One Wants to Give Us the Good News

We imagine that giving up pleasure foods demands a colossal massing of willpower. Thank goodness that's not true. If it were, I'd be in big trouble! The good news is that it's actually *easier* to give up the junk than to keep eating it. When we decide not to let a particular food past our lips ever again, we effectively shut the door on the egoic mind, the source of impractical food thoughts. Hence, to stop cravings, we need to turn away from thoughts about the foods we crave.

"That's easier said than done," you may counter, particularly when we're talking about physically addictive foods like sugar and chocolate. And I might have agreed with you before I gave up sugar and chocolate and found out how easy it was.

When we keep eating nonfood, we make it so hard on ourselves! But if we decide that a food like chocolate is no longer in our lives, we may miss it for a day or two, but then we forget about it—no pain, no feeling of deprivation. On the other hand, when we go on a diet and expect to be able to eat our coveted foods again on the maintenance plan, we end up counting down the days until maintenance time arrives.

If thoughts arise about a food that you've given up, simply ignore them. Don't, I repeat, *don't* give them an audience. If you spend a lot of time entertaining your thoughts about that food, you'll torture yourself. Give up the food for good, commit to not spending any time thinking about it, and life will be so much more pleasant.

The Upside: You're Not Really Giving Up Anything!

Given all the trouble that pleasure foods create in terms of disease and overweight, it's clear that our bodies weren't designed to eat them. If you think of it that way, it's easier to eliminate certain foods. If you're still resisting this change, though, because it's hard for you to imagine yourself eating primarily nutritious foods, it's totally natural. Don't worry about it. Just keep reading.

Abstinence sounds draconian from the perspective of a pleasure eater. It's a leap of faith, something that can only be experienced after you make the commitment to no longer give a certain addictive food a place in your life. Abstaining from addictive foods makes you feel better and is much healthier, but if you're someone who eats just for pleasure, like I did, it might be hard to believe that you won't be missing out on something.

However, what you can't really know until you've put abstinence into practice is that *you're not really giving up anything.* You're just establishing a different relationship to food, one that's more wholesome, freer, and less obsessive. The reason abstaining from pleasure food works is because you don't eliminate the pleasure of eating; you simply *eliminate eating food solely for pleasure.* That's a big difference. Even if you eliminate all of your favorite foods (and I'm by no means suggesting you do that), you'll still get pleasure from eating because food tastes good, and even healthy food is pleasurable to eat.

But I'll Feel So Deprived!

"But I'll feel so deprived that I'll go crazy and eat everything in sight!" you may be thinking. The bulk of current diet wisdom tells us not to ever let ourselves feel deprived because if we limit ourselves, we'll overeat later. We have tons of evidence to support this idea right in our own diet repertoires! We go on a diet, give up our favorite pleasure foods for a time, and then, when the diet ends, we go wild and eat them until our stomachs hurt.

The truth is that you can't continue to eat whatever you want, particularly the addictive foods, if you want to be free from your challenging relationship with food. You've done that, and you know it doesn't work. By not depriving yourself of these foods, you're trying to appease the Child so that she doesn't cajole you into eating everything that's not nailed down. But when you align with the Wise Witness, you recognize that the Child is using the idea of deprivation as a ploy, and you learn to stop listening to her. In this way, you break free from your conditioning rather than trying to manage it.

Try asking yourself, "What is it that will feel deprived if I give up an addictive food—my body or me? Is it true that my body will feel deprived? Or is it truer that I'm fantasizing about having a certain taste experience?" The truth is that the body won't feel deprived, the ego will. The Child will. Deprivation is a conditioned idea that the Child has talked to us about so many times that we've actually come to believe it. The Child tells us that we're feeling deprived, so we deserve two slices of chocolate mousse cake and a hot fudge sundae. She uses the idea of deprivation as an excuse for overeating, and we comply. The body, on the other hand, couldn't care less. It eats whatever is in front of it.

Deprivation is a conditioned idea that tells us we should be able to expect certain taste experiences because we've had them in the past. If we're used to having dessert, we come to expect it, and when we don't have it, we tell ourselves the story of "being deprived" and get in a tizzy about it.

The body isn't deprived without dessert. It needs a certain number of calories; vitamins and minerals; and a healthy balance of protein, carbohydrates, and fats. If we're giving it these things, it's not deprived.

Deprivation is a lie that the Child tells you. It's how we characterize the Child's tantrum when her desire for pleasure food is not being met. Once you see this, you're on to the ego's game, and you can't be tricked into believing in or following the lie. You're no longer attached to getting pleasure from pleasure food. When you're free from that attachment, you still enjoy food as much as, if not more than, before, but *you no longer need to get pleasure from a particular food at a particular time.*

You Can Still Have Treats

In transitioning to healthier foods, it's helpful to identify a few foods that you don't have an addictive relationship with that you consider treats. Find foods that you don't want to keep eating and eating once you start. If, at any point, you discover that you can't stop eating them, eliminate them—that is, if you want to be free of the addictive relationship.

When I want something a bit more interesting than protein, grains, and fruits and vegetables, I eat: low-fat, baked blue corn chips; small amounts of cheese; brownies that I make using bananas and carob instead of sugar and chocolate; popcorn; toasted whole-wheat pita pockets; peanut butter; raw almonds; frozen fruit (grapes, dark sweet cherries, oranges, bananas); dried, unsweetened apples or pears; or muesli that I make myself. I can eat these foods in moderation because they don't make me feel out of control.

How do you know whether you can have just a little bit of a treat food? If you can set a rule for yourself about it and stick to it, then it's a treat food you can moderate.

You Can't Keep Eating the Same Things

People tell me, "I'm so tired of suffering, just tell me what to do and I'll do it." But when I suggest eating differently, giving up the junk, giving up food that has no nutritional value, food that we can't stop eating and in all probability were never designed to eat, people make a beeline for the door. "I'll do anything you want, but don't ask me to give up the food I love. Don't get between me and my food, and no one gets hurt."

You can't leave out the food component and expect to lick this issue. Sure, it would be nice to think that we could take off the weight and then eat whatever we wanted. But that's a pipe dream.

Those in the food industry aren't fighting fair. They design foods that are irresistible and, as much as we would like to, we can't moderate these foods. If we could moderate, we would have. We have to stop engaging in the kind of thinking that keeps us on the dieting, gaining, dieting treadmill. The costs to our self-esteem and our health are huge! Aren't you ready to stop this way of living?

Eating as Much Bread as I Want Isn't Freedom

Growing up, I loved eating out because restaurant meals meant an unending supply of bread and butter. Hard rolls were my favorite. Winding my way to our table one night out, I spied hard rolls adorning the place settings. I was ecstatic! Even before the waiter came to take our order, I asked him for more rolls. I asked him so many times that the poor guy finally gave up and brought me a giant bowl of them. In retrospect, this may have been meant as a dig at my gluttony, but I couldn't have been happier. I dug in, and ate my fill.

We think that choice is freedom, but the opposite is actually true. For people who are overly involved with food, *choice is bondage.* When I make an eating plan for myself, it may be true that I've eliminated spontaneity. But I've also eliminated the gut-wrenching internal debates over "Should I or shouldn't I indulge?" and blocked the Child's access point. If my decision is already made, she doesn't have a chance to sneak in and steer me toward the wrong foods and eating too much.

Being able to eat whatever we want and as much as we want is a common fantasy. It's brought to us by none other than our good friend the Child and, surprise, surprise, it leads us in the direction of suffering. Imagining that other people get to eat whatever they want and not gain weight, we get jealous and decide we've been dealt a lousy hand in the card game of life.

But let's follow this idea through to conclusion. Imagine that you can eat as much junk as you want and stay thin. Here's what would happen:

1. By playing out this fantasy, you're eating mostly junk, and there is no off switch for that stuff. The defining characteristics of junk are that it's not satisfying and you can't stop eating it. As a result, you're overfilling your stomach and feeling bloated, lethargic, and uncomfortable most days.

2. Junk has little or no nutritional value. You're not giving your body the nutrition it needs, so you are becoming increasingly unhealthy.

3. If sugar is in the mix, you're experiencing mood swings, and the people around you aren't about to award you any popularity prizes.

4. Finally—and this is a big one—you feel out of control around junk. Of course, you may counter, "So what if I feel out of control? I can eat as much as I want, remember? That's the whole point of this fantasy." But feeling out of control around food is no fun. There's no freedom in it. It doesn't feel good to be addicted to a substance and not be able to stop consuming it.

There you have it: the whole picture of getting what we thought we wanted. Like all other desires that come to us courtesy of the ego, this one is empty and brings suffering. Being able to eat as much junk as we want is the booby prize!

The Weight Loss Starts!

Weight loss is a tortoise and the hare race. There are no brownie points for being quick off the starting mark. Instead, it's about going the distance and getting a body that you'll like for life, not just for a few weeks. You probably already know how the hare does things because you've been hare, done that.

Here's how it might have gone down: You went on a diet, lost your excess weight quickly, loved your new body at the end of the diet, and then, faster than you shed them, you started piling on the pounds again. It's natural. When you finished the diet, you were excited about getting to eat all of your favorite foods again, and you went overboard. Then it was back to "Hello, chubby!"

Cementing the Second Step, Wise Food Choices, helps you avoid this pitfall. Everyone is different, so start to make changes in your diet in a way that feels right for you. Remember, you're creating a lifestyle change, one that you'll keep for the rest of your days. Your reward for making this change is twofold: 1) a healthy body that stays at a natural weight and 2) freedom—you won't have to struggle and suffer over feeling out of control around food.

The first step is to eliminate foods you haven't been able to moderate or, at the very least, not let them into your house. Know that when you eliminate something, it's out of your life for good. You can't be wishy-washy about it or it won't work. Once you cut one thing out, you'll see that it's not difficult to do. When you eliminate something, you stop thinking about it, which means you stop desiring it, and you don't suffer. Desire equals suffering. When you don't completely eliminate a food from your diet, you don't banish it from your thinking. And thinking about food is where all the trouble starts.

I can promise you one thing: if you screw up your courage and take the plunge, as scary as it may seem and as resistant as your Child might feel about this prospect, *abstinence will prove a truly easy, stress-free solution*. Here are two strategies for abstaining from pleasure foods:

1. *If you're a big junk-food eater, start by eliminating one junky item.* For example, if you like having a Coke, fries, and a cheeseburger for lunch, start by cutting out the fries. (In the beginning, don't sit near someone who's eating them if you can help it!) See how this feels. You might miss fries for the first few days, but then notice how easy it is *not* to eat them. If a thought about fries arises, ignore it. Don't pay attention. Think about or do something else. Pretty soon you'll notice that you don't even think about them anymore.

    Once you discover how easy this is, try eliminating the next item. When you feel ready, move on to the Coke. And after that, try eliminating the whole category of fried foods.

    You don't have to make these changes overnight. There's no hurry because we're talking about a new way of eating for the rest of your life, a new relationship with food, not just a diet.

2. *Cut out most, if not all, of the junk.*

    This strategy makes most sense if you are not a big junk-food eater. I was able to take this step because, at the time, the only real junk I was eating was sugar and chocolate.

If you're beginning to heal your food addictions, it's very possible that you're already starting to lose weight. In the first year after I gave up sugar and chocolate, I lost 10 pounds without even trying! One reason this can happen is that you may find that the foods available to you after you give up your addictive foods are a little less sexy and, therefore, harder to overeat.

Don't worry, though, if you haven't started to lose weight yet. Everyone is different. The next chapter, which introduces the Third Step, Wise Eating, will help you see lower numbers on the scale.

Negative Beliefs about Eating Nutritious Foods

Let's move on to your beliefs. Here's your chance to uncover any negative beliefs you may have about eating mostly healthy, nutritious foods. You may be surprised to discover your beliefs about making wise food choices. As you read, circle any that ring true for you.

What Eating Nutritious Food Means about My Character

- ✾ I'm a cold fish.
- ✾ I'm no fun.
- ✾ I'm holier than thou.

What It Means to Others (Friends, Family, Colleagues)

- ✾ They'll think I'm:
  - ○ Arrogant.
  - ○ A party pooper—no fun to be around.

  - Someone to envy.
  - Someone they love to hate and gossip about.
  - An example of how not to live.
  - Too perfect.
- They won't want to be around me. I'll lose all my friends, and even my family won't want me around.
- I'll maintain a normal weight. Because I look different, my friends will feel awkward around me, like they don't know me anymore.

What It Means about How I Live My Life

I eat to nourish my body, and that means:

- I'll be miserable.
- I won't experience pleasure in my life.
- My body will maintain a stable weight range, and I'll blow all my money on clothes.
- I'll become vain and superficial.
- I'll lose my heavier friends because they'll envy me and won't want to be compared to me when we're together.
- I'll stop socializing. People won't want to be with me because I'm no longer using food as entertainment.
- I'll stop dieting for good, and that means I won't be able to relate to my friends who are always dieting.
- I'll be lonely.

What It Means about My Ability to Be in Relationships

I eat to nourish my body, and that means:

- My body will come to its natural weight, and that means:
  - I'll get unwanted sexual attention.
  - I can't hide out anymore.

- ○ I'll feel self-conscious.
- ○ People will want things from me that I won't want to give.
- ○ I won't attract the kind of partner I want because potential partners will only want me for my body.

What It Means about My Career

I eat to nourish my body, and that means:

- ❀ People at work will view me as superior and stuck up.
- ❀ I'll lose out on promotions.
- ❀ I'll never live up to my potential.

Inquiry for Resistance to Wise Food Choices

This section is pivotal to healing. It's your chance to take the beliefs you've uncovered to inquiry, a powerful tool I discovered by studying *The Work* by Byron Katie. Inquiry helps you see that what you've been believing is the root of your food and body-image suffering. Inquiry is the Perry Mason of evolution. If, like Perry, you put these pesky beliefs on the witness stand to see whether they hold up under cross-examination, they'll end up in jail, not you.

Ultimately, no matter how much you dress it up, food is nice-tasting fuel. It's the stuff we stick in our tanks to keep the body moving, thinking, working, playing, and breathing. However, as we've seen, this basic truth about food has done little to prevent us from forming wildly romantic beliefs about it and creating an overblown relationship with it. Now that you've explored a wide range of ideas about your body and food, you're ready to take them to inquiry.

Are the painful, negative beliefs you circled true? Whether you admit it or not, you've been living life as though they are. I've come to see that no single thought is big enough to hold the whole truth. At best, a thought is a partial truth, a single perspective. If we have enough presence of mind and detachment from our thinking to question whether a negative thought is true, we can diffuse its power. The power a thought has over us is only the power we give it. *Chances are that if you're suffering, you're believing a thought that's not true.*

Go back to the food beliefs you just circled and any additional beliefs you might have discovered, and take as many of them to inquiry as feels right. Ask yourself these two questions about each negative belief:

1. Is it true?
2. Is the opposite as true or truer?

If the negative belief is not true, think of some examples to support the positive, opposite belief. Here is what your inquiries might look like:

Negative Belief: Eating mostly healthy food means that I won't enjoy eating anymore. I'll be miserable.

Inquiry:

1. **Can I know beyond a shadow of a doubt that this is true?**
2. **What is the opposite of this belief?** Eating healthy foods means that I *will* enjoy eating, and I will still experience happiness and pleasure in life. **Could this be as true or truer than your original belief? What is your evidence for this?** I can't know how healthy foods will taste to me after my taste buds readjust. It's very possible that I will enjoy eating as much or even more than before. The bottom line is that I can't know the future. There are plenty of times when I'm engaged in what I'm doing and enjoying myself without food—like when I go for a walk on a nice day or listen to great music. I know that my life can still be pleasurable without the experience of eating certain foods.

Negative Belief: Junk food is my only source of pleasure.

Inquiry:

1. **Can I know beyond a shadow of a doubt that this is true?**
2. **What is the opposite of this belief?** Junk food is not my only source of pleasure. **Could this be as true or truer than your original belief? What is your evidence for this?** Just being alive is pleasurable! I get pleasure from seeing a sunset, taking a hot bath, reading a good book, sleeping soundly, listening to music, and doing things that are aligned with my life purpose. There are so many ways I get pleasure other than by eating junk food! If junk food were my only source of pleasure, I would be happy to sit alone and just eat. But I don't do that. I eat while I'm watching TV or reading. In fact, I never just eat! If junk food were so special, I wouldn't need to entertain myself while I eat.

Wise Food Choices Check-in

Phew! You made it. You got through the Second Step. Now be honest, was it really that bad? Piece of carrot, right? What I mean by "you got through it" is that you read about and are considering making some of the changes I discussed. Perhaps you are beginning to introduce more whole, healthy foods (those that are grown) into your diet and eliminate some junk food.

Don't be discouraged if your diet isn't healthy yet. You have a history with junk food that probably spans many years, and some of those foods are emotionally tied in. The Second Step might take months or even years to fully complete! Take whatever time you need to create this new lifestyle. It's not a race. It's a new way of eating and living that brings you freedom and peace of mind, not to mention a healthier, slimmer body.

Although the steps are sequential, it's okay to move on to the next chapter and begin working on the Third Step while you continue to work on the First and Second Steps. But before you do, please take a moment to read the following Chapter Summary and tick off the appropriate items on the To-Do List. Refer back to them often as you continue reading about the next three steps. This will reinforce the information and keep it fresh in your mind.

Chapter Summary

❑ Food is grown, not made.

❑ Food delights all five senses.

❑ We're programmed to love food.

❑ Eating pleasure foods has trained our taste buds to desire them.

❑ Eating mostly fast or processed food has meant that we've been choosing taste over health.

❑ We put a tremendous amount of emotional and mental energy into our relationship with pleasure foods.

❑ The double whammy is eating junk and skipping healthy, nutritious foods. The cost of the double whammy is that the body misses out on the nutrition and it has to expend energy to get rid of the junk.

❑ Listening to the body doesn't work if you're eating the wrong foods because they throw off your taste buds and your body's signals for hunger and satiation.

❑ When you give up all junk, there are still plenty of healthy foods that you can use as treat foods.

❑ When you stop eating junk, your taste buds change, and the healthy food tastes better than the junk ever did, but without all of the negative side effects.

❑ To stop wanting junk food, stop eating it.

❑ It's much harder to keep eating addictive food than to stop eating it.

❑ If you're addicted to a food and can make a rule about it and stick to it, you can keep eating that food.

❑ You can never be free of an addictive food by eliminating it temporarily. If you hope to eat an addictive food again someday, you'll continue to fantasize about it.

❑ If you decide to abstain from a food, you can't be wishy-washy about it.

To-Do List

Check off the tasks you've completed:

❑ I created a list of pleasure foods.
❑ I asked myself the following questions about each one:
  o Does the prospect of eating this food make me feel giddy?
  o Does it have little or no nutritional value?
  o Am I satisfied with eating one bite or does this food always leave me wanting more?
  o Do I feel out of control around it?
❑ If I answered yes to any of those questions, I limited or eliminated the food.
❑ I handled my addictive foods by either:
  o Finding a strategy I could stick to around them or
  o Eliminating the food for good.
❑ I limited or eliminated a junk food.
❑ I limited or eliminated most junk food.
❑ I made a list of foods that are no longer in my life.
❑ Most of my calories now come from healthy, whole foods that are grown.

CHAPTER 4
The Third Step: Wise Eating

• ◆ •

In the last chapter, you learned about what to eat. Now it's time to learn *how to eat.* Sorry, what did you say? You can skip this chapter? Okay, I get it. If you didn't already know how to *eat,* you wouldn't have the eating and weight issues that led you to pick up this book in the first place. Eating is a skill you already have in spades. Understood. But do you already know how to eat wisely?

Wise eating is learning to eat from a place of presence, balance, and calm rather than from a frenzied, out-of-control, mechanical, or can't-get-enough-of-this-heavenly-substance-called-food place. If you put the Third Step into practice, you'll adopt new ways of eating that will guide the course of your weight loss and serve you well for the rest of your life. It will teach you how to first recognize and then neutralize the Child's tricks that sabotage your weight loss, while deftly dodging the Critic's whip as she tries to flog you into shape.

If you're well versed in the subject of body weight and diet, some suggestions here may not be new to you, but please keep reading. You may learn a few surprising things, including how current practices and advice keep people stuck in their eating patterns.

Prior to developing the Five Steps, I thought I knew everything about this subject, but there were gaping holes in my understanding.

I was still struggling with my weight because I didn't have the right tools—the wise eating tools—to heal my issues.

If stressful thoughts come up while you're reading about wise eating, be sure to jot them down and question them in the inquiry section. Also, to stay on track with the wise-eating suggestions, remember to tick off the items that apply to you on the checklist at the end of the chapter. If you do those things, you'll be well on your way to making the Third Step your own. Good luck and have fun!

Breaking the Trance

Many of us go "zombie" when we're eating and become oblivious to how much food is going in. Without knowing it, we shovel in food like we're the Energizer Bunny set loose in a carrot patch. Anything we can do to become aware of and interrupt this pattern is helpful.

Personally, I like to stand up and walk around a bit. If I'm at a restaurant, sometimes I go to the ladies' room, even if I don't need to, just to break the trance. Another helpful strategy is to put your fork down between bites. When I go unconscious, I can get into a pattern of loading up my fork for my next bite while I'm still chewing the previous one. To counteract this tendency, I stop, put my fork down, and take a few breaths before continuing with my meal.

If you tend to race through meals, it's easy to overfill your stomach. It's amazing how many calories can go in when you're eating fast! Make a conscious effort to eat in slow motion and chew your food thoroughly. This is especially important when you're very hungry. Otherwise, the Child can get the upper hand and say, "I'm hungry. It's time to let loose and eat a lot!" When you're shoveling rather than eating, you can't enjoy your food nearly as much.

A Closer Look at Emotional Eating

In the second chapter, I gave you wise-thinking kung fus to combat emotional eating. Here are some behavioral tools to complement your king fus. First, make eating a sitting-down activity. Eat with your tush in a chair and your food on a plate. Why? If you study your emotional eating habits, my hunch is that you'll discover that emotional eating often happens when you're standing up.

When a strong emotion sends you racing toward the fridge, it's not like you're going to take the time to prepare a three-course gourmet meal, silver service and all. The scene probably looks more like "frantic clawing at the half-eaten, leftover piece of coffee cake in the fridge" or "shoveling gooey spoonfuls of Dulce de Leche straight out of the container using fingers."

There's a certain level of denial in this behavior. It's as if we're saying to ourselves, "If I cram the food down fast enough, maybe I won't notice how much I'm eating. And, best of all, I won't have to fully experience this uncomfortable feeling. I'll anesthetize myself with food to avoid the emotional discomfort."

Another possibility is that your emotional eating takes place in the car. Imagine that you've just had a gut-wrenching conversation with your spouse or boss and you're motoring home with snacks in tow. Here, Superman's got nothing on you. Able to deftly tear open packages with a single hand while steering with the other, you are Super-emotional-eater!

My point is that emotional eating happens in a hurry. We eat out of the fridge or pantry or over the sink or in the car when we're possessed by the "emotional-eating crazies." Neatness and etiquette fall by the wayside. Expediency is the priority. If you take the time to sit down and put your food on a plate, though, it helps you wake up and be more conscious of what you're doing.

Pretending Not to Eat

You can eat a lot of food when you're not paying attention. The Child tricks you into believing that if you're not paying attention, what you're eating doesn't count. So you believe that calories that come from nibbling don't count. But they do.

For a long time, I had a habit of eating while talking on the phone or cooking. I spend a lot of time on the phone, and because I do most of the cooking in our family, I'm always in the kitchen, I'm always on the phone, and I'm always cooking.

I was so accustomed to nibbling while I did these things that it took a lot of practice to create a new, non-nibbling habit. To change this pattern, I needed to see the truth—that on some level I was pretending that I wasn't eating. Because nibbling isn't a meal, I wasn't noticing it as much. I also wasn't losing weight. I'd reduced my calories, but because I didn't include nibbles in my calorie count—probably because I couldn't keep track of them all—my excess pounds stayed stubbornly in place.

The other thing about nibbling was that it robbed me of eating pleasure. Because my attention was divided, I couldn't completely enjoy the food or focus on my phone conversation or my cooking. And that was ultimately unsatisfying. To finally overcome this habit, I decided not to nibble for one day, just to see if I could do it. Then one day turned into two days, and so on. Why not give this a try? See if you can go one full day without nibbling.

Just Eat When You're Eating

If food has been your drug of choice, you've used it to numb out. That's been your habit. To get free, you need to create a new habit of being present during the experience of eating—to *just eat when you're eating*.

It's rare for people in our culture to just eat—we're usually either driving, watching TV, talking on the phone, having a conversation, or reading while we eat. But sitting down and experiencing each mouthful of food as it leaves our fork? Now that's radical!

See if you can stay awake while you eat. I'm not talking about not nodding off and falling into your soup. I'm talking about staying present and experiencing the sensations of eating rather than escaping into thought.

Whenever I just eat without doing anything else, I notice that the Child says, "This is boring." She wants to rush the experience and distract me from what's happening in the moment. When it comes right down to it, she isn't interested in the sensory experience of eating at all—she only wants us to eat if we can do something else at the same time.

For the ego, the problem with being fully present when we're eating is that it brings us into the moment. The sensation of eating, like any other sense experience, is a portal to your true self. Biting into an apple involves all five senses. If you bring your awareness to the sensations of eating, you can't help but be in the moment, aligned with your true self instead of the ego. And if you're out of the ego, you don't need it, and it's out of a job.

Rather than repeating the experience of numbing out according to the ego's plan, try turning the tables on it. Let the experience of eating become a new way of aligning with your true self and strengthening your connection with it. *Just eat when you eat* for a meal or a snack at least once a day.

Losing Weight Using Reasonable Portions Rather than Listening to Your Stomach

To maintain a healthy weight, we need to educate ourselves about portion size. The truth is that *the portions we imagine we can eat are much larger than what we can actually eat without gaining weight.*

Restaurants have contributed to this misunderstanding. To get a leg up on the competition, they started offering larger and larger portions. As a result, we've been conditioned to expect them. But it comes as no surprise that eating large portions means gaining weight.

Find out what portion sizes are appropriate for you rather than accepting the heaping platefuls restaurants dole out. Do you know about how many calories you need to maintain a healthy weight? If you don't, consider working with a nutritionist to find out. Once you have an idea, translate that number into food choices and portion sizes. You can pick up a pocket calorie counter at your local bookstore or supermarket to help you with this.

For example, find out what the portions look like in a 400- to 500-calorie meal and use that as a guide to help you eat more reasonable amounts. If you go to a restaurant, look at the portion you receive. Is it reasonable? If not, don't eat it all. Only eat the amount of food that you decide is appropriate.

If I know a restaurant serves large portions, I either split my order with someone or ask the server to bring a smaller serving. When I receive a larger portion than I need, I push the excess to the other side of my plate or transfer it to another plate during the meal and then take it home in a doggie bag.

Assuming we can rely on our stomach to tell us how much food to eat is one of our main misconceptions. Judging from the feeling in our stomach after we've eaten a reasonable portion, we often think we're still hungry, so we eat more. But the feeling of satiation doesn't register right away after we've eaten, and for some people, it never registers.

There are different degrees of hunger. If you're tummy-rumbling hungry, that's a trustworthy sign that it's time to eat a meal. But when you've already eaten, using *the feeling in your stomach* to tell you how much more to eat or when to stop *is an unreliable gauge*. Sometimes the more we eat, the hungrier we feel!

If the body were good at telling people when to stop eating, there wouldn't be so many obese people around. Although the sensations in your stomach might be a gross measure of whether you're hungry enough to eat a meal, they don't tell you when to put on the brakes. *Let portion size, rather than the feeling in your stomach, determine how much you eat.*

Hungry? Thirsty? Stressed? Tired?

In the midst of an uncomfortable sensation, many of us look to food to feel better. Rather than asking ourselves what we actually need in the moment, we make a beeline for the fridge. We insert food and then wonder why we don't feel better. Innocently, we thought we'd addressed the body's need or the uncomfortable emotion, but find that we're right back where we started.

At one particular *Skinny Thinking* Workshop, many participants told me that when they were about to reach for food, they tried asking themselves if what they were feeling was truly hunger. Surprisingly, they realized that often they were actually thirsty or tired instead. Afterwards, they wondered how many times they'd mistaken thirst or fatigue for hunger in the past.

Stupefying as it may seem, food doesn't solve every problem. We've trained ourselves to cope with uncomfortable sensations by eating, only to find that the food made us feel worse than ever. By overfilling our stomachs without addressing our true physical or emotional needs, we're expecting food to give us things it was never designed to provide. It can only numb us momentarily, postponing the inevitable return of an uncomfortable sensation or emotion.

Just for the heck of it, the next time you think you're hungry, ask yourself, "Am I hungry right now? Or is it possible that I'm thirsty, tired, upset, or excited instead?" When you're about to reach for food and it's not time to eat, question whether you're really hungry, or if you're experiencing some feeling of emptiness or discomfort. You'll be amazed at how many times food isn't what you want after all.

Making Friends with Hunger

Okay, I can see you bristling at that headline up there. Relax. I'm not asking you to subsist on a celery stalk and a lemon wedge. I have no interest in you being ravenous and miserable from now on. And I know that few other words in the English language evoke more fear than "hunger." We're used to seeing it flanked by equally scary words, like "pestilence," "famine," "disease," "starvation," and "death." No wonder it evokes such a visceral response in us!

Hunger avoidance is built into many cultures. In Judaism, people wish each other well by praying that their children never know hunger. In most societies, ascending the socioeconomic ladder and landing in the cushy land of wealth and prosperity means never having to worry about hunger. The ironic thing is that by shunning hunger, many people have ended up compromising their health.

Sellers of fad diets reinforce this hunger phobia by stirring it up and then reassuring us that their diet tames the hunger beast. "Have no fear," they boast, "on this diet you will never feel hungry." Because I'm all about telling you the truth, even if it's not what you want to hear, I'm telling you that *this type of advice does you no favors*. To maintain a natural, healthy weight, we need to learn to tolerate some hunger before we eat a meal.

If that's the case, how do we deal with our fear and resistance toward it? Before we dive in, let me clarify. When I say "hungry," I don't mean "cannibalizing your neighbor" hungry. I'm talking about the slightly uncomfortable, tummy-rumbling sensation that you feel when your stomach is empty. Many of us have forgotten what hunger even feels like, equating it with not being full anymore. That isn't hunger, it's just not feeling full.

Hunger is a good friend who's been given a bad rap. If you let it, it can help you end your weight battle for good. See whether it's possible to welcome some hunger and allow it to be there for a short time rather than sprinting to the fridge the minute you notice you're no longer full.

Our Fears and Beliefs about Hunger

Conditioned to be afraid of hunger, we avoid it at all costs, exaggerating its discomfort way beyond the reality of the experience. As a result, many of us never let our stomachs get empty. Checking in with our stomachs several times a day, we act quickly to fill the slightest void.

Maintaining a normal body size means learning to live with some hunger, and not being willing to embrace hunger means living in a heavier body. If you're not comfortable with this idea, look at your beliefs about it. Perhaps you're giving hunger more meaning than it warrants. Does it stir up fears that you're not going to survive?

Begin by abandoning the notion that *you know* about hunger. Get curious about experiencing it. Welcome it and see what it actually is, as opposed to what you think it is.

To help your unconscious ideas surface, ask yourself why hunger is so frightening or uncomfortable. What are your beliefs about it? What will happen if you let yourself get hungry? On a separate sheet of paper or in your journal, list your fears and beliefs. What are the meanings you've given hunger? What stories do you tell yourself that cause you to reach frantically for anything edible to immediately quell any hunger sensations?

Here are a few I've come across in my travels:

- ✿ If I let myself get hungry, my blood sugar will drop, I'll get shaky, and I won't be able to function.
- ✿ If let myself get hungry, I'll eat everything in sight.
- ✿ Hunger is too uncomfortable. I can't bear it.
- ✿ It's too scary. I can't let myself go there.

Let's take a closer look at each of these notions:

- ✿ *If I let myself get hungry, my blood sugar will drop, I'll get shaky, and I won't be able to function.* I'm not talking about extreme hunger that impacts your energy level or blood sugar. I'm talking about allowing yourself to experience a natural physical sensation that's cueing you that your body is ready to eat a meal.
- ✿ *If let myself get hungry, I'll eat everything in sight.* This is a story you've told yourself to keep yourself from seeing the real truth about

hunger. It may be true that you've let yourself get very hungry and have then overeaten in the past, but again, I'm not talking about that crazy, chew-your-own-hand-off kind of hunger. Hunger and overeating don't have to go together unless, of course, that's what you believe and you turn it into a self-fulfilling prophecy.

❀ *Hunger is too uncomfortable. I can't bear it.* Is that really true? Or are you imagining a scary future and tying it to your concept of hunger? Try letting go of your assumption and allowing yourself to get hungry. See what happens.

❀ *It's too scary. I can't let myself go there.* Ask yourself, "What am I afraid of? Is it starvation? Is it discomfort? What is so frightening about letting myself experience hunger?"

Now it's your turn to see what hunger really is rather than living according to your uninvestigated ideas about it. I'm throwing down the gauntlet. I challenge you to devote a day to experimenting with hunger by allowing yourself to get hungry before each meal or snack. Each time you feel a hunger sensation, ask yourself, "Am I hungry?" When you're hungry, wait 30 minutes or an hour before eating. When you do this, you may notice that the hunger comes and goes, and the most uncomfortable feelings don't last. If you ignore them and don't fill them with food right away, they turn into other sensations that are easier to live with. At some point, hunger sensations level off or even disappear rather than getting worse and worse.

After your day of experimenting with hunger, compare your experiences with the fears and beliefs you listed earlier. Were your negative assumptions about hunger true?

Comfort and the Ego

It was 12:30 p.m. and I had two thoughts in quick succession: "I'm really hungry" and "I won't be able eat until 2:30." I felt disappointed and worried about whether I could hold out until then.

But as soon as I accepted the fact that I wouldn't be able to eat until later, a miraculous thing happened—I forgot all about food. In fact, I didn't give it a second thought until 2:30, when I was able to eat. Even more miraculous: I didn't feel hungry. I was engaged in what I was doing, and somehow the hunger sensation turned off.

Without thought, there was no sensation. I started to wonder: Which came first, the sensation or the thought? Had I really been hungry at 12:30, or did I look at the clock and think, "Hmm…12:30. Lunchtime. Time to be hungry now"?

I'll let you in on a little secret: The ego is always seeking comfort. The prospect of discomfort, no matter how small, sends it scurrying for the exit. Hunger is no exception. The ego says, "Why should I experience the discomfort of hunger if I don't have to? Life throws me enough curveballs already, but hunger isn't one of them. I don't *have* to feel hunger, so I'm not gonna!"

But, have you ever considered that hunger might be an aspect of the divine plan, integral to the optimal functioning of the body? Like eating, resting, and exercising, perhaps bodies need to experience hunger to run well. Could it be that hunger is how the body supports us in maintaining a healthy size?

Forget health for a moment and consider pleasure. Now that I have your attention…have you noticed how delicious food tastes when you're hungry? Even a carrot tastes like manna from heaven. When you allow yourself to get tummy-rumbling hungry, you enjoy your food in a way that isn't possible when your tank is full. When you're not full, but not quite hungry either, the taste of food and the experience of eating are not nearly as satisfying.

I've learned to actually like feeling hungry. (Don't fall over now. It's true!) I just like the way food tastes better when I let myself get hungry. I especially like the results of having allowed myself to be hungry: being thin and feeling energetic and light on my feet.

I've gotten into the habit of feeling hungry at various times of day, so it's not a problem. It's a normal part of my life. And if I can't eat when I'm hungry, that's not a big deal, either. I know I'll get around to it eventually. *The fear is gone.* Food will be there for me at some point. I don't have to manage the feeling in my stomach or check in on it constantly.

Think of your body like a car. You don't indiscriminately pull your car up to the gas pump. When you see the fuel gauge getting close to empty, you start looking for a gas station. In the same way, check if your stomach tank is genuinely empty before you fill it. Ask yourself if you're really hungry. If not, wait until you feel the growling in your stomach that means the body needs food. This sounds simple, yet most of us rarely wait for that signal. If you're serious about having a more balanced and sane relationship with food, begin to live with some hunger and wait to eat until you feel it.

The Exception

Although the general rule of thumb is to eat only when you're hungry, there is a qualification: Eat only when you're hungry, and *only if it's also when you've decided that you will eat.* If you've been overeating on a regular basis, it's important initially that you not follow the dictates of your stomach because overeating has thrown off your appetite, and it needs to readjust before you can trust your hunger. Your stomach sensations are unbalanced in proportion to how unbalanced your relationship is to food. You may think, "But I'm so hungry," but you've trained your body to be hungry frequently by feeding it often. In this case, it's helpful to come up with an eating plan that provides a reasonable number of calories, spread throughout the day, and use it as your guide.

Replacing Negative Thoughts about Hunger with Positive Ones

While you're experimenting with hunger, notice the thoughts that arise. If the thoughts are negative, does their magnetism pull you toward the refrigerator? If so, it's only natural. Our conditioning regarding hunger has been so overwhelmingly negative that it's natural to feel compelled to fill any voids with food.

One of the easiest ways to release negative ideas is to replace them with positive ones. Here are some positive thoughts to help you counter the ego's negative commentary:

- Hunger is good.
- Hunger is normal.
- Hunger is helping me reset my taste buds and my metabolism.
- Hunger is easy to tolerate.
- Hunger is healthy.
- Hunger is welcome here.
- Hunger is freeing me.
- Hunger is helping me to reach a healthy weight.
- Wow! I experienced hunger and I lived!
- My body is designed to get hungry before it eats.

More Wise Eating Habits

You Don't Lose Anything by Forming New, Healthy Habits

In the ego's world, there is always duality—pleasure seeking carries within it the seed of pain. The ego doesn't tell us that, of course, because we would be less likely to follow a promise of pleasure that also leads to pain. So it tries to hook us with the pleasant half of the story and avoids the unpleasant half.

The truth is the truth, though. If you want to maintain a natural, healthy weight, you can't keep your old habits. You can't continue to eat the same foods you've been eating and not monitor portion size. Let me repeat so this is crystal clear: You can't ever go back to eating what you've been eating. You can't ever go back to not monitoring portion size. You can't ever go back to eating when you're not hungry. Thinking you can return to your old habits is the kind of deluded, egoic thinking that has kept you yo-yoing over the years.

Accepting this truth and following your true self's impulses toward health and balance have no cost, no downside. In creating new, healthy habits, you don't give up anything. The pleasure is there as much as ever, if not more so, because there's no inner conflict. Not only will you reach a healthy weight, you'll get to keep your new body without struggle or worry for the rest of your life. It's a win-win.

Parties: To Eat or Not to Eat

If food has been your primary source of pleasure, parties can be a huge challenge. At a party, everyone is in a festive, devil-may-care mood, food and drinks are flowing, and people are busy meeting, greeting, and gabbing. How do you stay present with all of this stimulation? What do you do when tantalizing cheese puffs, chips, and mixed, salted nuts beckon? How do you keep the wise, rational part of you in charge? What's in the Wise Witness's arsenal to fortify you in the face of these powerful temptations? Two words—a plan.

A plan can be as simple as "I will limit myself to healthy food and reasonable portions." It can be something you pen the day before or commit to five minutes before you leave for the party. Plans put the wise part of you in charge and keep the Child at bay. The Child will fight you on this because she doesn't like to commit. She'll say things like, "What if I want a few cheese puffs? What's wrong with that? Why do I have to plan that? Can't I just eat like a normal person?! Is this how life is going to be? I'm going to have to *plan* everything from now until I die?!" Ignore her.

One of the truths we uncovered about pleasure food is that it's hard to stop eating it once you've started. Therefore, if you can create a rule to establish a reasonable portion—and stick to it—by all means, allow yourself some cheese puffs. The bottom line is: Either limit or abstain from pleasure food unless you've decided to let loose and entertain yourself with it, and then eat it only if you're willing to accept the consequences of that choice.

Here are two suggestions for making a party plan. I've found that the first one is easier to implement.

1. Decide ahead of time that this party is not an eating event for you. Either eat ahead of time or plan to eat afterwards. I find that it's best to have eaten ahead of time because when you're surrounded by sexy nibbles, it's much easier for the Child to gain the upper hand and say, "What the heck! I'm going to eat because I'm hungry!" if you are, in fact, hungry.

2. Decide ahead of time to eat at the party, but to eat only the foods and portions that you designate. You may not know what will be served, but there are often crudités or a salad available, so you'll probably have some healthy options. Put your food on a single plate and limit your party eating to only what is on that plate—that food and nothing more.

With this trusty plan arrow in your quiver, you're ready to go forth and fend for yourself on the treacherous battlefield called the party. Forewarned is forearmed.

The Scale: A Great Weight-Loss and Maintenance Tool

Contrary to the advice in many books on eating and weight issues, it's okay to take your bathroom scale out of storage. I used to be afraid to weigh myself because I didn't want to know the truth. If I suspected that I'd gained weight, stepping on the scale would wreck my day. If I'd lost weight, I'd overeat to compensate for the unexpected boon and suffer over that! There was no way to win. For me, the scale was always either the harbinger of bad news or the impetus for bad behavior.

The ego doesn't want us to weigh ourselves because it doesn't want to know the truth. This is not only how it deals with food and weight—but with all of life! It wants to pretend it can do whatever it wants without accountability, and the scale represents nothing if not accountability.

How often should you weigh yourself? Weighing in once a week is probably okay for most people. You can make yourself crazy if you try to weigh in too often. And weighing yourself after haircuts and nail clippings is definitely over the top! Everyone is different, though. If you're cutting your calories by 200 per day and losing one pound a month, it's probably best not to weigh yourself more than once a month. For most of us, though, weighing in every week is fine.

"What about the jeans test?" you ask. If it works for you, keep doing it. The problem with using the fit of your jeans to monitor weight, though, is that jeans shrink after washing and stretch after wearing, so the results vary. The jeans test leaves room for doubt and, my, how the ego loves wiggle room!

After you reach a natural size, continue to weigh yourself so that you *know*, rather than speculate about, how much you weigh. That way, the pounds can't creep back on surreptitiously. If you don't let yourself gain more than a couple of pounds over your ideal weight before you do something about it, you can maintain your weight without stress or worry. You'll avoid going very far overboard with food again because you won't want to experience the consequences when you step on the scale.

Why a Plan Is Helpful

Imagining how food tastes is a slippery slope that leaves you vulnerable to backsliding (going off the plan you've made for yourself). When you imagine how something will taste, you create a desire for it. It's dangerous. Once a desire is generated, it begs to be fulfilled.

When you plan what to eat for the day, you eliminate the option of imagining and fantasizing about other foods, so desires for those foods aren't created. You also eliminate desire for what you are going to eat. If you know what you're going to eat, there's nothing to desire. You can't desire what you already have because *desire comes from wanting what you don't have.*

The ego resists committing to a plan with all its might. It's wishy-washy. "*Maybe* I'll do this," it says, or, "*I'll try* to do that." The problem with this approach is that it, too, leaves you vulnerable to backsliding because you didn't *really* commit. Whenever you notice you're unwilling to commit to a plan you've created, that's the ego trying to sabotage your intentions to eat well.

"What if I can't commit?" you may counter. "What if I'm in situations where I can't plan, and I'm forced to accept the food that's available?" Simple. As soon as you know what's available, create a plan within those parameters. You can say to yourself, "Okay, here's what's available. I don't have to put every food I see on my plate just because it's here. I can pick and choose what and how much to eat." If you just start eating without thinking about what you're doing or creating a plan, you start to slide down the slippery slope.

The Wise Witness isn't afraid of commitment. Here's how she deals with going out to eat: "We're going to a restaurant, and they serve buffet style, so I'll have a fist-sized portion of protein and fill the rest of my plate with vegetables. I'll eat that, and only that, and not return for seconds."

And here's how the Wise Witness might plan for a trip: "I'm traveling, and I need to bring enough food to last the 18-hour journey, so I'll eat X at this time and Y at that time." Or, "I'll be driving all day in an area that only offers fast food, so I'll bring healthy food with me. That way, I won't have to eat food that's not good for me."

You know that you can commit, plan, and strategize because you've done it many times when you've dieted. You simply ignore the Child, who always wants to thwart your plans. When most of us go off a diet, however, we let the Child start guiding our eating again. That's why we regain the weight we lost. The Child hates eating pragmatically; she always wants to be free to do what she wants, when she wants.

If you're having trouble committing to a particular food plan, your thoughts might go something like this: "What if I commit to eating X and then I find that I don't want to eat X? What if something else looks better? What if food is available on the plane and I'd rather eat that? What if I'm still hungry after I eat what I've allowed myself? I don't want to be limited."

That's just the Child talking. Notice it and calmly ask yourself if that's what you want to follow this time. What has following this voice gotten you in the past? Recall situations when you didn't plan or commit. What have you done in those situations? Have you been able to eat healthy food in reasonable amounts or have you overeaten? What's your track record?

A Thought Diet

A thought diet is a truly transformational diet. It involves giving up certain kinds of thoughts about food, such as "Hmm, what would *taste yummy* right now?" It stops us from romanticizing food, which is crucial, because the moment we start fantasizing about how a food would look, smell, or taste, we create desire and desires demand fulfillment.

For many of us, the pattern of indulging our food fantasies has become our default position. Once the fantasizing gains momentum, though, it's like trying to stop an oncoming freight train. There's almost no way to stop it once it gets rolling.

Planning can help you jump-start pragmatic thinking and put the kibosh on these kinds of romantic food thoughts. If you stop thinking about food romantically, your relationship with it will change and so will your weight. *You can change your romantic relationship with food by learning not to think about it or to think about it pragmatically.*

If you have a food plan and you find yourself thinking about food that's not on it, turn away from those thoughts. If you have a set menu for the day, there's no room for food fantasies, only for functional thoughts like "Okay, these are the two options and this one makes sense." This way of thinking about food frees up your mind for other pursuits. It also becomes easier the more you do it. When you find yourself starting to fantasize about a food, stick to your thought diet and focus on something else.

Reprogramming the Taste Buds

When you start eating more nutritious food, cutting out junk, and letting yourself get hungry before you eat, you discover that *healthy food starts tasting so much better!* That's because your taste buds become reaccustomed to the flavors of the nutritious, whole foods the body was designed to eat. By allowing yourself to get hungry before you eat, you help your taste buds along in this process. Because healthy foods are satisfying and don't cause you to overeat the way pleasure foods do, you tend to eat them in moderate amounts. As you begin to retrain your taste buds, jot down a few thoughts about what it's like to eat healthy foods now that you are restricting pleasure foods. What did the carrot or orange taste like? How did you feel afterwards? Were you satisfied or did the healthy foods leave you wanting more?

Losing Weight from the Ego versus Your True Self

Remember the Dreamer back in Chapter 1? That's the aspect of the ego that keeps you locked in a fairy tale. When you're identified with the Dreamer, the hope of being admired motivates you to diet, and keeps you on a diet by spinning fantasies about the kind of life you'll lead, the clothes you'll wear, and the partner you'll attract in your new, svelte body. If you fall off the wagon, look out! The Critic will be right there, calling you every name in the book for going off your diet. The Critic uses moral judgments about food, along with browbeating, to keep you on a diet, while the Dreamer motivates you with the lure of desire fulfillment. (The Child, of course, tries to keep you eating pleasure food the whole time.)

Your true self, on the other hand, encourages you to bring your body back into balance by prioritizing health, freedom, and happiness.

Your true self moves you to change your diet permanently rather than go on another diet temporarily. If you're aligned with your true self, you see the whole picture about what food can and cannot offer you—and what a thinner body can and cannot offer you—rather than deluding yourself about how great life will be after you lose weight. You live in the present moment and remember that your ultimate goal is freedom from the conditioning that has kept you suffering.

Exercising from the Ego versus Your True Self

To the ego, exercise, like dieting, is a means to an end, a strategy to get a sexy body that it thinks will bring admiration and success. Other than that, the ego has no use for it. Just as it's perfectly happy to go on unhealthy crash diets to get a sleek body, the ego has no compunction about jumping into a punishing exercise regime rather than building up to it slowly with health in mind.

Your true self, on the other hand, values nourishment and self-care, and delights in the feeling of being alive. Noticing that your body's energy is waning, it sends a message urging you to rest or sleep. Seeing that your body would benefit from movement, it plants the idea of going for a walk. It actually enjoys the feeling of exertion and well-being that comes from moderate exercise.

Yo-Yoing in Smaller Swings

Many of us who've used food for comfort and entertainment have gone on one diet after the next, each time hoping to solve our weight problem for good. Our closets have become mini-boutiques to accommodate the skinny, medium, and heavy versions of our bodies. If yo-yoing has been your pattern, as your thinking comes into balance and your eating naturally follows, your weight might continue to swing for a while.

Over time, though, the size of the swings will gradually diminish. For example, if your weight used to swing by 30 pounds, it may swing by 20 pounds, then by 10, then by 5, then by just 1 or 2 pounds. Keep in mind that most people can't go from swinging by 20 or 30 pounds to 1 or 2 in a short period.

If you're still yo-yoing, you may think you're not progressing, not healing. But healing is a process, not an instantaneous fix. The key is patience. Don't torment yourself if you find that your weight continues to go up and down for a while. It's natural.

Backsliding

Changing your eating habits can take a long time because it involves so many areas of your life. You have to change not only your relationship with food, but your grocery-shopping habits, your cooking habits, how you respond to your environment, and how you interact with the people you spend time with. Be patient with yourself and don't beat yourself up if you backslide.

Dissolving Resistance to Wise Eating

Take a moment now to notice any resistance you feel to wise eating. What stressful beliefs have you unearthed while reading about or adopting these new habits regarding food, portion control, planning, and weighing yourself? Write them down, and question them. Take a look at the following sample inquiries. If these two thoughts resonate, answer the questions for yourself.

Negative Belief: I'll never lose weight this way! It's going to take forever!

Inquiry:

1. **Can I know beyond a shadow of a doubt that this is true?**
2. **What is the opposite of this belief?** I will lose weight this way and it won't take forever. **Could this new belief be as true or**

truer? **What is your evidence for this?** I can't know the future. Hence, it's true that I can't really know if I will lose weight this way or how long it will take. However, if I'm doing the math right, if I'm eating healthily and reducing my portion sizes or calories, I'll inevitably lose weight.

Negative Belief: I'm a failure because I'm not implementing the first three steps perfectly.

Inquiry:

1. **Can I know beyond a shadow of a doubt that this is true?**
2. **What is the opposite of this belief?** I'm a success because I'm not implementing the first three steps perfectly. **Could this new belief be as true or truer? What is your evidence for this?** I know that the author did plenty of backsliding and she healed her relationship with food. She wrote that we don't have to do this perfectly to heal. I'm making an effort to change my thinking and my old habits and this means that in spite of backslides, I am a success and will heal.

Wise Eating Check-in

Phew and double phew! You made it through the Third Step. How does it feel? Are you still breathing? Is your heart still pumping blood? You've absorbed some very challenging information and, hopefully, have begun to eat more wisely. Congratulations on making it this far!

Chapter Summary

- ❑ Many of us go "zombie" when we're eating.
- ❑ Nibbling calories count.
- ❑ Nibbling while doing other things is not very satisfying because your attention is divided. You can't fully experience eating or whatever else you're doing.

❑ Most people have a skewed idea about the portions they can eat and still remain at their desired weight.

❑ Planning eliminates imagining and unconscious eating.

❑ To know when to stop, pay attention to calories or portion size rather than your stomach.

❑ Weighing yourself regularly helps you keep your weight within a healthy range.

❑ Hunger is your friend.

❑ If you let yourself get hungry before you eat, you won't have a weight problem.

❑ Hunger is not a reliable gauge for when to stop eating.

❑ To lose weight, you have to consume fewer calories than you're using.

To-Do List

Check off the tasks you've completed:

❑ I've been more aware while I've been eating.

❑ I waited to eat until I was hungry.

❑ I asked myself whether I was hungry, thirsty, stressed, or tired, to avoid eating when I wasn't really hungry.

❑ When I was tired, I rested rather than reaching for food.

❑ I chose how much to eat based on portion size rather than satiety.

❑ I ate more slowly.

❑ I put my fork down in between bites or walked around during a meal to interrupt my automatic food shoveling.

❑ I *just ate* when I was eating. I ate by myself, concentrating on the experience of eating.

❑ I was able to *just eat* rather than doing other things at the same time.

❑ I sat down to eat and put my food on a plate.

❑ I avoided nibbling.

❑ I created a plan.

❑ If I deviated from the plan, I didn't beat myself up.

❑ I've been weighing myself regularly to help me manage my weight.

❑ I let myself experience hunger for a day and compared the actual experience to my fears and beliefs about hunger.

❑ I've been waiting until my tummy talks to me before eating.

❑ I would like to lose weight, and I have been cutting out _____ calories per day or reducing my portions.

CHAPTER 5

The Fourth Step: Wise Living

• ◆ •

Congratulations on getting the first three steps under your belt. Let's take a minute to recap. Have you been starting to incorporate the steps into your life?

The First Step: Are you beginning to see the whole picture of food and let go of your romantic fantasies and misconceptions about it? Are you thinking less about food, thinking about it mostly when you're hungry or when it's time to eat? How are your kung fus for cravings and emotional eating coming along?

Don't get discouraged if you're finding it difficult to put these new habits into practice. Looking for fulfillment and relief by way of pleasure food has been your pattern. Repeating it has strengthened and reinforced it, so it's not surprising that it takes time and practice before you're able to make a new choice. But have no fear. You'll be vying for your kung fu black belt in no time!

The Second Step: Is your diet getting healthier? Have you found a strategy that allows you to continue to eat your addictive foods? If not, have you been able to abstain from them? If you decided to abstain, have you been surprised by how easy it's been?

The Third Step: Are you waiting until your tummy rumbles before you eat? Are you eating more slowly and bringing more awareness to your eating? Have you been weighing yourself regularly? When you are about to enter a social eating situation, have you remembered to create a plan?

What about backsliding? Have you backslid? If so, it's to be expected—it's a natural part of the process. It certainly *doesn't* mean that you've fallen off the wagon and won't heal. If you've made it this far, you're definitely on Recovery Road. Healing may not happen on the ego's timetable, so remember to be gentle with yourself and let it be okay to make mistakes.

Permanently healing eating issues is a maturation process. There's a part of you that hasn't grown up yet. Once it begins to mature, there's no turning back. When sixth graders write book reports, they don't have to strain to remember how to form the letter "f." That knowledge already lives in them. It's the same way with the Five Steps. Once you've learned them, you may backslide occasionally, but that knowledge will stay with you.

Now that you're coming out of denial, seeing the truth, and changing your old habits, you can never go unconscious again. Following the Five Steps develops that part of you that never grew up in relationship to food; you become the wise parent and align with your true self. When you've dieted in the past, the diet book took on the role of the wise parent. But after the diet, if you hadn't changed the way you thought about food, your relationship with it never had a chance to mature and you've been stuck repeating the same pattern ever since. This is your chance to change it for good. Now, on to the Fourth Step!

If you have a love affair with food, it means that you're using food to satisfy needs that it was never designed to fulfill. This is a happiness issue. When you're not feeling happy, it's natural to go after pleasure food, hoping to trade your current experience for one you think you'll like better. The Fourth Step, Wise Living, is an opportunity to explore how the way you're living and expressing yourself might be keeping your natural happiness from you. It's a chance to learn why you feel you need to look for pleasure from food.

If you're fighting with people, castigating yourself, or afraid to ask for what you want or to say no, the ego has you locked up, and will keep you racing to the fridge faster than a roadrunner on steroids. Fighting strengthens the ego: peace aligns you with your heart. If you want to stop eating your feelings, reducing your reactivity to others can be a great help.

Improving your communication skills can help you accomplish this and at the same time create adaptive, positive relationships. In the upcoming pages, you'll learn ways to express how other's actions impact you, discover what you're repressing, and reduce or even eliminate confrontations.

Everyone wants to be happy, but not everyone tries to get happy through food. Ask yourself what seems to be missing for you? How are your relationships? Is your life the way you want it to be? Do you wake up excited to see what a new day will bring? If you're not happy because the structures in your life don't suit you and your relationships aren't harmonious, it's going to be hard to change your eating habits because you're using eating as a crutch to manage your unhappy life. Instead, why not take steps to change your life by beginning to arrange it to support your happiness?

Once you start to make these changes and see through any conditioning that's been blocking your joy, you align with your true self. You learn a new way of being, living, and expressing yourself from your heart. Putting this step into practice pays dividends in all areas of your life.

Living from Your Heart

Wise living means living from your heart. This may seem antithetical. I've spent the last four chapters teaching you how to align with the Wise Witness, and now I'm doing an about-face and telling you to live by the fickle, unpredictable whims of the heart? Let me explain.

In our culture, we teach people that the best way to live is to follow their rational mind. We laud analysis and thoughtful, well-considered choices and actions. Of course that's the way to create a happy, meaningful life. Isn't it?

The truth is that when we make choices from our head, they're often fear-based, arising from a defensive posture that mistrusts life. Following our head means following the ego's strategy, which often involves finding ways to keep a scary, imagined future—that we have zero evidence will ever manifest—from showing up on our doorstep and devouring us along with whatever semblance of a life we've managed to create.

Living from the heart means choosing to follow something else. It means getting quiet and following a subtle, intuitive knowing that moves you to do what you love and what you're good at. It means asking, "What would I really love to do? What sounds like fun?" and then arranging your life accordingly.

The Critic thinks this is the stupidest thing it's ever heard. "Living that way, you'll fritter away your days being a dilettante. What kind of teaching is this? You're an adult now and you should be a responsible and productive member of society! After all, what would happen if all the grown-ups just decided to throw caution to the wind, let loose, and have fun? You have responsibilities and people relying on you!"

I'm not suggesting that you suddenly start listening to the Child. The Child goes after pleasure following ego-based desires. These are all trumped up, don't deliver, and ultimately lead to suffering. Instead, I'm recommending that you live from your heart, align with your true self, and move toward what truly feels good and is fun for you.

Try to remember what it felt like to be very young, delighting in life and in new and wondrous experiences. Learn how to live this way again by asking yourself, "What makes my heart sing? What do I enjoy and get excited about doing?" Then follow the insights and impulses that arise. You're meant to be happy in this life!

Connecting with a Fulfilling Life Purpose

Finding a fulfilling life purpose is learning how to live so life feels like an adventure. It's turning work into play. All people have to do things they don't want to do, but no one has to do work they don't like.

In order to stop wearing a path to the fridge, connect with a life purpose that actually engages you and feels fulfilling, something that you love and are good at. When you're so excited that you can't wait to start a task, food becomes less interesting and sexy. You're in the flow, and no ego pleasure can compete with that high. From that place, food is simply fuel. It tastes good and you enjoy it, but you're so engaged in what you're doing that you can forget to eat, and only a gnawing stomach reminds you to stop and take a break.

Human Doings

Because our culture tells us that happiness is something to be attained rather than something to be noticed, we've become a society of doers. We *do* rather than *be* because we've been taught that doing will get us what we need in order to have a meaningful and happy life. Once we've gathered the external trappings of a successful life, we think we'll be happy. Yet when we're too focused on doing, we miss out on our natural happiness. In addition, because we do too much and don't value feeding our souls enough—going within, resting, being quiet, listening, and meditating—many of us are perpetually stressed out.

Ask yourself, "Is there a part of me that feels happy and at peace in this moment?" How connected do you feel with it? That is your true self. The more you rest in that part of you that is always content, the less identified you are with the ego, and the less you will look to things outside of yourself for happiness.

If you aren't happy, it's because you're telling yourself an unhappy story, you're doing too many things, or you've made choices that are not aligned with what you love to do. Your mind can cause you to be unhappy because minds are, by their very nature, negative. For example, your mind could be telling you that what you're doing isn't meaningful or that you're not doing it well enough. So, it's possible to be living a life aligned with your life purpose but still not be happy because your negative mind saps the joy out of it. The mind declares, "This is how things should be and how you should be...but you're not. You're not doing it right."

In our culture, we associate eating with celebration and parties, so when we think our lives lack enjoyment, we try to create fun through food. The happier we are, the less likely we are to create a painful, out-of-line party with food, like the one I had after my dance recital. If we're aligned with a fulfilling life purpose and we let ourselves rest more, ease up on ourselves, and allow ourselves time to just be, then our whole life feels more like a party, and we don't feel the need to create one with food.

Pushing

Your true self allows what is unfolding in life, intuits what is true in the moment, and moves in that direction. The ego, on the other hand, has an agenda and pushes until it gets what it wants. Pushing your way through life blocks happiness. Have you noticed? It's such hard work!

For example, the ego might push you to work at a job that you don't like out of fear. "You won't be able to pay your bills if you leave this job," it says. "Wait and see. If you leave it, you'll be living on the street."

Pushing yourself, even when you're doing what you love, will cause you to become out of balance. Do you have a habit of pushing, pushing, pushing until you either exhaust yourself or get stressed out? Notice where that line is and take a break, even a short one, when you hit it.

When we push ourselves beyond what we want to do, we're apt to try to make it up to ourselves through food. Grown-ups unwittingly introduced us to this habit by offering treats to us as kids when we cleaned our rooms or got a shot. Now, we offer treats to ourselves when we push beyond what we really want to do.

When the joy goes out of what you're doing, stop, even if it's just for a short time, and pick it up later. And by all means, if you are working at a job you dislike, don't just keep doing it. Tell yourself the truth about it. Try to find ways to be able to do what you want to do instead. Take steps to move in that direction rather than organizing your life to avoid what the ego fears.

Feeding Your Soul Instead of Your Stomach

Just because thoughts and feelings enter our awareness doesn't mean we have to act on them—we can just *notice* them. Being aware of thoughts and feelings rather than merging with them and acting on them is a huge leap forward in our evolution, not to mention our ability to make peace with eating, weight, and our bodies.

If you stop turning to food for comfort, you need to replace that relationship with something else. That something else is your own true self. You connect with it when you spend time doing your "9's" and "10's" and take time to feed your soul.

In addition, make it a point to move into the thought-free state as often as you can. Each of us spends time in the thought-free state every day. We just don't know it. The thought-free state is that instant when you're looking at a gorgeous sunset and your mind stops. Then the thought "Oh, what a gorgeous sunset" arises and takes you out of it. Any time our attention is on sensation—what we are seeing, hearing, touching, smelling, or tasting—and we're not caught up in thoughts or feelings, we're in the thought-free state. In these moments, we dive between our thoughts and align with our true self. You can rest in the thought-free state when you're waiting in line, walking to your car, or even folding your clothes. All you have to do is notice that you're thinking and ask yourself, "Where's the quiet?"

You're always being fed from your deepest self, your true self. Acknowledging that and choosing to make the time to stop and experience it helps you heal and grow. The next time an unpleasant emotion arises, notice it, allow it to be, and then ask to receive insights and healing. *Noticing moves you out of thought.* Ultimately, freedom from any eating issue is about becoming more established in your heart. To do this, make the time to be quiet sometimes, and choose not to be in a lifestyle that's so busy and stressful that you're constantly getting lost in thoughts, emotions, and doing.

When you feel the urge to experience some pleasure from food, but are not physically hungry, try this exercise that helps you move into your heart:

> *Imagine yourself moving from your head (the ego's world of thoughts, emotions, and cravings) into the space of the heart. You're floating downward into a delicious, peaceful space: the velvety black cave of the heart. Here, nothing is required of you. You're free from the stresses and problems of daily life. Simply rest here for 5 to 10 minutes and recharge your batteries. Pick a certain time each day to devote to this practice.*

As you practice moving from your head into your heart, you will weaken your cravings by strengthening your connection to your true self. The more you practice, the more resting in the cave of the heart during your day will become second nature.

Wise Responding

Wise living also means learning to respond to others while remaining balanced and aligned with your heart. This can be especially challenging when another person is angry and confronting you. When you're being attacked, it's natural to want to attack back. This only creates an argument. Instead, begin by acknowledging the other person's perspective and empathizing with them.

My husband and I have learned to use four words that immediately diffuse a charged situation and keep me from reaching for food. If one of us is upset, the other tries to respond with, "I can see that." These words alone can be enough to create a reprieve so that we can catch our breath and relate to each other from our hearts. By saying "I can see that," we acknowledge the other person's perspective, they feel heard, and it's easier for them to move back into their own heart.

When you speak to other people, try to see where they're coming from, to imagine how you would feel if you were in their shoes. Ultimately, all acts of hostility and abuse arise from a hurt place in the perpetrator. Though it may be difficult to see at the time, these aggressive acts are actually cries for love. When people are acting out of the ego, acknowledge that and know that it's not who they really are. Remember how awful it feels to be so contracted and have compassion for their suffering.

Tread lightly with yourself here and don't expect to instantly be able to put this habit into practice. Just remember, when someone is angry, they're coming from the ego, so try not to get hooked or escalate the situation.

Other People's Criticism and Aggression

There is no such thing as a nice ego. Whether it's ours or someone else's, the ego is mean and ruthless. Some egos can put on a nice face to get what they want, but they're never purely altruistic. When people are aligned with their ego and acting out its nastiness, it's natural to move into the same negative state. We're conditioned to take others' negative behavior personally and react by attacking, defending ourselves, or stuffing down our feelings. These responses keep us aligned with our own egos.

Moving away from someone else's ego that wants to fight is far from easy. Your own ego is likely to be breathing down your neck, saying things like, "Are you just going to stand there and take that from him? You wimp! Where's your backbone?" The other guy's ego is egging you on and in cahoots with yours. Both are trying to push, dare, and shame you into the fray. If you have the presence not to fight, all the better, because this is a battle you can never win.

A better response to somebody else's negative behavior is to not react at all, and stay aligned with your true self instead. That requires only one thing: that you realize that the other person is in the ego and that egos egg other egos on. Once you understand that, you can choose to step back, notice what's happening, and *not take the bait!*

Not taking the bait is a huge evolutionary step. A sage once said, "It is easy to be enlightened in heaven." Well, it's not as easy to be enlightened in the hell created by a bully or someone who's taking his or her foul mood out on you, but it's well within your power.

It's Just Conditioning

If you're able to notice when conditioning has been triggered, either yours or someone else's, you can learn to sidestep your emotional-eating response. Miracle of miracles, you can even catch an emotion before it's been created!

When people are criticizing you, it's just their Critic talking—not who they are. Although there may be a sliver of truth in what they're saying (that is what hooks you), because they're speaking from conditioning, you know that their words can't contain the whole truth. When people criticize, judge, attack, or blame, in that moment, they believe their conditioning and they're suffering. The best relationship you can have to them is one of compassion.

Being able to respond with compassion when people are attacking us only requires being able to see the truth—that their behavior doesn't reflect who they really are. It's just their conditioning talking. If you can be present enough to recognize conditioning instantly when anger is coming at you, you won't have time to take it personally, and there will be no upset. You already know how hard it can be to regroup once you're upset, so the next time someone criticizes you, try saying to yourself, "That's just conditioning." Your noticing it will preempt your impulse to take it personally. Then, no negative belief has a chance to arise and subsequently create messy negative emotions.

Whether conditioning is coming at you from the inside or the outside, the approach is the same. Notice it right away, label it as conditioning, and don't buy into it. That way, you can sidestep both the emotion and the emotional-eating response.

Speaking Your Truth

From an early age, many of us created emotional connections with sweet, salty, or fatty foods, using them to medicate ourselves when we were afraid, angry, or sad. Now, as adults, rather than uncovering the painful beliefs that underlie those emotions and using inquiry to dissolve them, or expressing what is appropriate to others in the moment, we stuff down our feelings with food. Eating might delay and blunt our reactions, but when we stuff our feelings with food instead of dealing with them, we may end up beating ourselves up or taking out our upset on those around us in passive-aggressive ways.

For most of my life, my fear of incurring the wrath of others was so intense that I would do almost anything to avoid it. As a child, I wasn't in mortal danger from adults, but they did have power over me. As I got older, my fear of other people's anger was way out of proportion to the actual threat it posed. No one was going to kill me, but the terror I felt was akin to what I would have felt if I were being chased by a grizzly bear!

I assumed that if I told people that I didn't like what they were doing or saying, they would reject, ridicule, or humiliate me. My fear of disappointing people and desire to please them were so great that they often kept me from expressing the authentic "no" ringing inside me. My fear turned me into a liar and manipulator to get the approval of others. I rationalized not speaking my truth as conflict avoidance and then judged myself for being spineless. In those moments, I didn't know whom I was angrier at, other people or myself. In my head, I would rail at them for doing whatever they were doing, and then I would blast myself for being unable to respond.

I identified with the Meg Ryan character in the movie *You've Got Mail* when she dreamt of coming up with the perfect put-down. In one scene, she finally comes face-to-face with her antagonist, and delivers a great, biting quip. To her amazement, the experience feels nothing like what she'd imagined. She feels awful because it hurt to hurt someone else, even someone she disliked intensely. This is the difference between speaking the ego's truth and speaking your truth from your heart. Speaking the ego's truth creates separation and makes everyone feel bad, and speaking the Wise Witness's truth brings people together and connects them to their hearts.

Wise Communicating

When we get upset, it's natural to want to lash out at whomever we think is responsible for our pain and, of course, reach for something tasty to eat. In a confrontational situation, your ego will urge you to settle the score by attacking the other person. Instead, try to find a place to be alone or at least away from that person for a while.

Notice that you're aware of the emotion, and acknowledge that, therefore, the emotion can't be you. You're not the anger or the hurt feeling. Dis-identifying with it in this way greatly diffuses it. Next, drop your story about the situation and focus on the body sensation associated with the emotion. Witness it, but don't feed it with more thoughts about how bad or wrong the other person is. Just experience the sensation.

After some time, you may notice the sensation beginning to shift or dissipate. Don't impose any timetable on it. Just give the sensation the time and space it needs. Once the feeling has dissipated, you have a choice: to let the other person know what's come up for you or to deal with the upset within yourself using inquiry. If you choose to speak to the other person, do your best to do it in a neutral, nonjudgmental way. Make factual observations and express the impact that the other person's behavior had on you without blaming. Here is an example from my life:

A friend and I had plans to meet. I arrived at the prearranged time and place, but my friend was nowhere to be seen. I waited for 10 minutes, and still no friend. When I called to ask her what had happened, she responded that she'd had a change of plans. This response upset me because:

1. *She changed her plans without letting me know.*
2. *I had to phone her to find out what was going on.*
3. *If I had known that she wasn't planning to come, I could have called someone else.*

Here are two possible responses, one that could lead to emotional eating and one that represents a more balanced approach:

Stuffing my feelings and pretending there is no problem:

I can stuff my feelings and pretend that it's not a problem. After all, I don't want to make her mad or make her think that I disapprove of her. If I tell her the truth, she may not want to be my friend anymore. I can tell her, "No problem. These things happen. It's fine. Don't worry about it."

Expressing myself in a balanced way (after any anger has subsided):

1. I can factually express the truth: "Sarah, we had plans, remember?"
2. I can express how her behavior impacted me: "If you had told me sooner, I could have invited someone else."
3. I can tell her what I want. I can let her know what I'd like her to do in the future: "Next time, please let me know ahead of time if you need to make a change."
4. I can let her know how her behavior has affected my feelings about the relationship: "Sarah, what you did makes it hard for me to stay open to you, and I want to let you know that I will be doing my own work on this as well."

Whether or not you include step 4 will depend on the nature of the relationship. For instance, it might not be appropriate to express those thoughts in a work situation.

Speaking our truth is healing, diffuses conflict, and actually brings us closer to others, while speaking the ego's truth separates, inflames, and escalates conflict. We know we are speaking the ego's truth when we find ourselves blaming, name-calling, globalizing (using words like "always" and "never"), and judging. In speaking the ego's truth, we act out and defend our conditioning; in speaking our true self's truth, we take responsibility for it.

By expressing impact, we're not asking the other person to change. Instead, our expression might take the form of asking for what we want in the future, e.g., "I'd appreciate it if...." This isn't the same thing as telling someone he or she has to change, which can sound judgmental. How we say things and where the words are coming from make all the difference.

When you acknowledge your weaknesses or admit you're having trouble releasing something, you know it's coming from your heart because the ego doesn't admit to its failings. Once you've expressed yourself from your heart, if you're still having trouble moving on, asking the other person for an apology can help. You can simply say, "It would really make a difference to me to have an apology. If that's something you feel you could do, I think that would help me feel better." Apologies move both parties into their hearts.

It takes a lot of practice and self-restraint not to attack and not to go for the pleasure food. If you tend to react immediately, changing this habit will require time, so be patient and gentle with yourself, just like you would be if you were teaching something new to a young child.

Repressing and Compulsive Eating

I had knocked myself out getting ready for my husband's homecoming— cleaning the house, the car, and our dog, buying flowers, and writing a nice card. I couldn't wait to hear his key in the lock, sure that he would be thrilled by all that I'd done. Soon after he walked through the door, he started playing with our dog. Crushed, I created the story "He loves the dog more than he loves me." His sweet kiss and embrace did nothing to undermine my story of being unloved and unappreciated. Rather than take my story to inquiry, I snubbed him, sulked, and stuffed my disappointment with half a container of muesli.

Compulsive eating stems from repressing feelings—usually anger—and may require therapy to heal. Everyone has repressed emotions. It only becomes a problem when they cause us to hurt others or to become self-destructive. In our innocence, we eat compulsively because we think that distracting ourselves from unpleasant feelings is the best way to take care of ourselves. We're uncomfortable and use food to create an experience that we hope will feel better. Instead, we end up eating self-destructively.

Compulsive eating is more frequent among women than men because, in our culture, it's less acceptable for women to express themselves and go after what they want. When we don't go after what we want, when we aren't true to ourselves, or when we don't express or stand up for ourselves, we get upset and repress our anger.

If making art is your passion, you may not follow it because you're afraid that you won't be able to earn a living as an artist. Or if you aren't cut out for parenthood, you may end up having children because of conditioning that says you should. If you follow your conditioning instead of your heart, you may end up living a life that doesn't suit you. Unless you change that, you'll continue to feel unhappy, repress your feelings, and eat compulsively.

Find Out What You've Been Repressing

To heal compulsive eating, find out what you've been repressing. Asking questions is like summoning your own fairy godmother—you powerfully ask for help and set the intention to heal. It's a courageous act that says, "Show me. I'm ready, already!" Take a moment and ask yourself the following questions: What am I repressing? What am I angry about? Is there anything I'm not doing out of fear or habit? Is there anything I'm keeping myself from saying? How do I avoid asserting myself? What am I afraid of? Simply allow the answers to surface in their own time.

Even if you discover an ego-based desire that you're not following, it's not healthy to repress it. Instead, let it see the light of day, acknowledge it, and then decide whether or not you'll follow it. Don't delude yourself into thinking it's not there because, if you do that, you'll find yourself in roadrunner mode again in no time flat. If you choose to pursue the desire, don't fret because even going after egoic desires can lead to growth and evolution.

Asking these questions demonstrates your willingness to see the truth about how you've been living. How are you not living your truth? How are you not speaking your truth? By asking rather than thinking you already know the answers, you're humbly admitting that you don't know. You're surrendering to your own higher wisdom and are asking to be shown the areas of your life that you are in denial about. In effect, you're lifting up the carpet of your life to discover what's been hiding under there.

After you find out what you've been repressing, take action. Do or say what you've been avoiding and set the intention to stop repressing your emotions in the future. Healing is one part excavation and one part relearning and retooling. If you want to stop stuffing yourself with Oreos at the next sign of stress, you've got to change how you're living, how you're responding to life's little (and not-so-little) hiccups. In this way, you will learn to break the habit of repressing in the first place!

Becoming More Assertive and Choosing How You're Spending Your Time

Another way to stop repressing is to become more assertive. If you feel that you're not entitled to say no or stand up for yourself, you will probably get angry and either repress or feed your feelings. When this happens, you're likely to eat at the same time that you're having an angry conversation in your head. You heal this pattern by expressing what you need to express from your heart and attending to the emotional issue that's come up rather than feeding it with food and more thoughts.

You might be afraid that people won't like you or that your spouse will leave you if you start speaking your truth, saying no when you mean no, or asking for what you want. When those kinds of fearful beliefs come up, record them in your journal and test them by taking them to inquiry. Then, ask yourself, "What's the worst thing that could happen if I express myself?"

Next, examine the structures in your life. If you're angry or resentful about the way your life is set up, you may need to make some changes. Stop doing things that you don't want to do, or at least take steps in that direction. Even though you may feel locked into your life, you don't have to spend most of your time doing things you don't want to do. To become empowered and stop repressing and eating your feelings, redirect your life so that you're doing what you love.

Unless you acknowledge that you're *choosing* how you spend your time, you'll feel victimized, angry, and resentful, and be much more likely to eat emotionally. Eliminate as many unpleasant tasks and activities as possible from your life so that you can be happy.

Often, we get going in the wrong direction because our minds or other people's minds tell us we *have* to do this or that to attain a certain standard of living or to survive. But if you're doing what you enjoy, you won't need to get happiness from things or from food.

Happiness

There are two kinds of happiness, the ego's version and real happiness, and they look very different.

In exchange for doing things you hate, the ego offers you a nice car or house or a big piece of chocolate cake as a reward so that you can feel good about yourself. But you don't have to get happiness from feeling good about yourself on an egoic level. When you're being true to yourself, you feel good because you genuinely like what you're doing. Then, feeling good isn't conditional. You won't need to be famous, beautiful, sexy, or rich to feel good about yourself.

If living your heart's truth or following your passions doesn't generate the money, success, or admiration the ego desires, then so be it. It takes courage to live simply, doing what you love instead of having all the niceties that other people think you need, but it can allow you to experience real happiness.

Healing Low Self-Esteem

An important part of living wisely is learning wise self-talk. Negative self-talk creates low self-esteem and, despite everything we've achieved, thoughts like "I'm no good" may still plague us. They will continue to do so until we begin to question, see through, and detach from them.

When we tell ourselves that we're lazy or lack self-control or anything else that's negative, we're acting as the ego's mouthpiece. In those moments, we rattle off negative self-talk as if it's actually true. Thanks to countless repetitions and reinforcement, we eventually come to accept this negative rap as a factual depiction of who we are, and we no longer question it.

Negative self-talk is like a witch's incantation: It's mesmerizing. To break the spell, you need a powerful antidote: awareness. Set the intention to *notice the way you habitually talk to yourself*. When you notice yourself falling under a spell and a negative feeling is on the scene, ask, "What am I telling myself to make myself feel bad?" This interrupts the pattern.

Remember, if a thought makes you feel bad, you can know that it's not true. Take any negative belief to inquiry and you discover that it never tells the whole truth. Just because you have a history of falling under a particular spell doesn't make it any less a lie. Once you see the lie, the spell is broken, and the negative self-talk no longer has any power over you. If those thoughts arise again, *either replace them with positive thoughts, question them using inquiry, or turn away from them altogether.*

Eating to feel better actually adds to the problem of low self-esteem by causing you to feel less attractive and worse about yourself. It's a vicious circle: Eating the cookies brings a fleeting, nice taste in your mouth and momentary relief from a negative feeling, but then you berate yourself for not having any willpower and not losing weight. Conversely, *not* eating the cookies gives you a chance to:

- See what you're saying to yourself that caused you to feel bad in the first place.
- Use inquiry to become free of the negative belief that caused the negative feeling.

Remember, changing a deeply entrenched pattern can take time. Please be patient and tolerant with yourself as you chip away at your old habits. Can you choose to behave differently—just for today?

What Your Beliefs about Food and Eating Mean about You

If we're overly involved with food, we tend to create a morality around food and eating. Abstaining from food and denying ourselves is virtuous and indulging is sinful. We feel great about ourselves when we've been good, and castigate ourselves when we miss the mark. Beating ourselves up for our lapses in willpower and telling ourselves that we're weak, we allow our eating and concern over how our body looks to dominate our lives. Here are some stressful things you may be telling yourself when you eat emotionally:

- I'm weak.
- I'll never get the body I want.
- I can't get on the right track in my life.
- I won't attract the kind of partner I have always dreamed of.

To help uncover your beliefs about food and eating, ask what you're telling yourself that's causing you to feel bad and reach for food. Keep a running list in your journal. Take each belief that feels true to inquiry.

Do I Deserve to Be at a Healthy Weight?

Recently, a woman told me that she'd been holding the belief "I don't deserve to be at my ideal weight." She balked when I reassured her that she did indeed deserve to have her body come back into balance. She asked, "Why is that? How could I know that it's true?"

I suggested that, rather than taking my word for it, she go inside and experience it for herself. I'm asking you to do the same. Move out of thought by using your senses. Focus on a sight, sound, or sensation. How does it feel? For me, it feels so good when I do this that questions of deserving or being worthy can't even arise. I immediately connect with a peaceful, happy feeling.

Your true identity *is* this good feeling of happiness, balance, and peace. In other words, there is nothing good that you don't deserve. When you move outside of thought, you can intuit the intention of your true self for both you and every other human being: health, ease, freedom, and balance. And if that is your true self's intention, there can be no questions of deserving or not deserving. Worthiness is a given.

The very idea that you don't deserve to be happy or thin comes from the Critic. When you understand this, you can immediately discount it. The Critic is a nasty piece of work, the aspect of the ego that generates all low self-esteem. So if you notice that you're feeling bad about yourself, you've bought into the Critic's rhetoric. See that for what it is, remember that the Critic is a liar, and ignore it.

Noticing that the Critic is on the scene will shift you back into the Wise Witness. From there, you will naturally experience well-being, and the concept of deserving cannot arise. When you're aligned with the

Wise Witness, there is no *you* left to deserve or not deserve. There is just a wondrous place of calm and joy and a melting back into a natural state of oneness. From there, the question "Do I deserve it?" is irrelevant.

Perfection

The perfection game was invented by the ego to keep us striving toward an imagined future that will bring everlasting happiness. The problem is that even if we achieve some of the goals that make up this dream, life never feels as good as we had hoped it would. It never feels completely satisfying.

The ego uses perfection to keep itself employed. It coyly assumes that if we stay focused on striving and the future, we will forget to notice the happiness that's already available to us. Being happy for no reason is our birthright. Happiness is always available to us and when we're quiet, when we stop thinking, we experience it.

The Critic thinks we need to have it all together to be happy, and the Dreamer imagines a future moment when we "arrive," when the years of work that we've done on ourselves finally pay off, and our dream of a "perfect me" comes true. According to the Critic, to get from our current, flawed "me" to the glorious realization of a "perfect me," we have to be vigilant, tyrannizing ourselves every time our humanness shows up. In other words, if we don't eat the way we planned to or if our body doesn't look just so, the Critic wants to make sure we castigate ourselves and make ourselves miserable. If we overeat or eat junk food one day, the Critic tells us that we've blown it and, after all we've done and tried, we've gotten nowhere with this issue.

But everyone can heal their eating and weight issues, even if those issues took a lifetime to develop. I'm living proof. It doesn't happen overnight, though. We progress, plateau, backslide, and then move forward again.

You don't have to get everything right to heal, and you don't even have to get to someplace called "100% healed." It's just the ego that

wants to be able to say, "I'm 100% healed!" or "Look how perfect my eating (or my body) is now." The salient question is whether your eating or weight are negatively impacting your health. If not, let it go. Why torment yourself? Ask yourself, "Is it okay for me to be human? Is it okay to be imperfect?"

If you answer no, you're really setting yourself up to be miserable. There's no such thing as a perfect person. Certain people appear to have it all together, but can we really know their experience? Can we know what their life feels like? Everyone's life has built-in challenges. Otherwise, how would we grow? Imagine how boring life would be without them.

One of those challenges, for those of us who strive for perfection, is learning to love and accept our human foibles, our imperfections. Can we learn to be tender with ourselves when we don't meet our own expectations? Knowing that life isn't easy, can we learn to be tolerant and loving toward ourselves? If we're going to try to perfect something, why not try to perfect being kind? Why not try to perfect being able to accept ourselves, especially when we let ourselves down or don't meet our own expectations?

Inquiry for Resistance to Wise Living

This section is pivotal to your healing. It's your chance to uncover more emotional-eating beliefs and take them, along with any stressful beliefs you might have about wise responding and wise expressing, to inquiry. Once you do, see what happens to your relationships with yourself, other people, and food. You think your beliefs are powerful? Questioning whether a negative thought is true—now that's powerful!

What Eating to Satisfy Emotional Needs Means about Me

In this section, circle each negative belief that causes you stress so that you can question it later.

What It Means about My Character

- I'm weak.
- I have no willpower.
- I'm a hopeless failure.
- I'm unlovable.

What It Means to Others (Friends, Family, Colleagues)

- I'm a loser because I can't get my eating under control.
- I'm an emotional wreck.
- I'm not living up to my potential.
- I'm someone to look down upon.
- I'm gluttonous.
- I'm an example of how not to live.
- My eating is:
  - Immoral.
  - Repulsive.
  - A turnoff.
  - Pathetic.

What It Means about How I Live My Life

- I'll never stay in a stable weight range and that means:
  - I'll stop socializing.
  - I'll stop trying to find a partner.
  - I'll feel like a failure.
- I'll always be on a diet, trying to get a handle on my weight, and that means:
  - I'll always be unhappy.
  - I'll always struggle.
- My weight will always yo-yo, so I'll never be able to maintain a normal weight.

What It Means about My Ability to Be in Relationships

⊛ I'll always be fat, and that means:
  ○ I won't be loved.
  ○ I'll end up alone.
  ○ No one will want me.

⊛ I won't be able to attract the kind of partner I want because I'll be judged for not being more together and in control of myself.

⊛ No one will want to be in a relationship with me because I'm always in a bad mood when I eat emotionally.

⊛ I'll never be able to reveal this shameful practice to my partner, so I'll always have to hide it.

What It Means about My Career

⊛ I won't have the respect of my subordinates, peers, or superiors.

⊛ People at work will think I'm weak-willed and lacking in self-esteem.

⊛ I'll lose out on promotions.

⊛ I'll take out my bad moods on my coworkers.

⊛ I'll never live up to my potential.

⊛ If I can't do a simple thing like manage my weight, I'll never amount to much.

These troublemaking beliefs are the root of your food and body-image-related suffering and now's your chance to address them. Take as many of them to inquiry as feels right, along with any stressful beliefs that arose when you were reading the Wise Responding and Speaking Your Truth sections.

For example, if the belief is "I'm weak," can you really know that that's true? The opposite of this belief is "I'm strong." This belief is at least as true, and it might be truer. "I'm strong because it takes great fortitude to move against the culture and prioritize health over taste. I'm strong because I'm reading this book. I'm strong because I have the courage to look at my relationship with food so that I can heal. I'm strong because I've been able to incorporate many of the suggestions in this book," you might say to yourself.

Here are two more examples:

Negative Belief: I'm a hopeless failure if I can't control my eating.

   Inquiry:

   1. **Can I know beyond a shadow of a doubt that this is true? What is the opposite of this belief?** I'm a success if I can't control my eating. **Could this new belief be as true or truer? What is your evidence for this?** I'm a success because I'm telling myself the truth about my eating. Only when I tell myself the truth about something can I learn and grow from the experience. If I were able to control my eating and I hadn't formed a romantic relationship with food, perhaps I would never be able to understand what food means to me or investigate and remedy what's really bothering me. I might miss the opportunity to tell myself the truth about what's going on and heal the conditioning that's robbing me of happiness.

Negative Belief: Speaking my truth means that my relationship with my partner will fall apart. Because I won't be repressing my anger, I won't be keeping the peace anymore, so we'll split up.

   Inquiry:

   1. **Can I know beyond a shadow of a doubt that this is true?**
   2. **What is the opposite of this belief?** Speaking my truth means that my relationship with my partner will *not* fall apart. In fact, it will get even stronger and more peaceful because I won't be

repressing my anger, so we'll end up staying together. **Could this new belief be as true or truer? What is your evidence for this?** I can't know the future, so it seems just as likely that speaking my truth will make our relationship stronger rather than tearing it apart. The very fact that I am speaking my truth rather than stuffing it with food will mean that I am likely to be happier and have healthier self-esteem, and that alone will make me a better partner.

Set a goal of taking at least one negative belief to inquiry every day. The more you question stressful thoughts, the less power they have over you, and the sooner they'll stop creating the negative emotions that move you to reach for food in the first place. So go for it!

Chapter Summary

- ❑ Wise living means acting and speaking from the heart.
- ❑ Make sure that you take time to do what you love to do, what you're good at.
- ❑ Take time to have fun and feed your soul. If the Critic thinks this is frivolous, remember—taking care of yourself is being responsible.
- ❑ Pushing comes from the ego.
- ❑ From an early age, many of us created an emotional relationship with sweet, salty, or fatty foods.
- ❑ Rather than stuffing our feelings with food, we can:
  - o Use inquiry to debunk our stressful thoughts.
  - o Stay present with our feelings.
  - o Express what is appropriate to others in the moment.
- ❑ Once we recognize that another person is in reaction or acting out of the ego, how we respond is up to us.
- ❑ When someone attacks us verbally, we're conditioned to take the behavior personally and react by either attacking back or

defending ourselves. Both of these responses strengthen the ego in us. Instead, we can choose to step back, take a breath, shift into the Wise Witness, and not take the bait!

❑ Speaking our truth could mean asking for what we want in the future (e.g., "I'd appreciate it if...").

❑ Telling someone to change, which can sound judgmental and angry, is different from speaking our truth.

❑ How we say things and where the words are coming from—the ego or the true self—make all the difference.

❑ Eating compulsively and bingeing both come from repressed emotions (particularly, repressed anger) and may require therapy to heal.

❑ Repressed anger comes from not going after what we want, not being who we are, not expressing ourselves in the world, not standing up for ourselves, or not doing what we're moved to do.

❑ Low self-esteem comes from believing negative thoughts about ourselves.

❑ When we have low self-esteem or feel bad about ourselves, we may try to feel better by eating. If we eat to get happy, it adds to the problem, causing us to feel worse about ourselves. It's a vicious circle.

❑ To reverse low self-esteem, replace your negative thoughts about yourself with positive ones.

To-Do List

Use this To-Do List to jog your memory as you put this new step of Wise Living into practice. Reading it over frequently will help you remember to begin to live more from your heart. This way of living supports your health, growth, and happiness, rather than reinforcing the pattern of emotional eating. Check off these items when you have been able to put them into practice:

❑ I noticed negative thoughts about myself arising and I replaced them with positive thoughts.

❑ I asked myself, "What am I repressing? What am I avoiding saying or doing?"

❑ I recorded the insights that arose and put them into action in my life.

❑ I spoke my truth to someone from my heart.

❑ When I felt wronged, I expressed impact from my heart rather than attacking.

❑ I said no when I might have said yes in the past and then felt resentful.

❑ I created a plan to rest more and not push.

❑ I created a plan to be able to spend more time doing what I love to do.

❑ I put making time for fun in my calendar.

CHAPTER 6

The Fifth Step:
Wise Relationship with Your Body

• ◆ •

Congratulations! You've made it through all of the steps that deal with eating and self-expression, and now it's time to heal your relationship with your body. Before we move on, let's do a quick check-in. How are you doing with the First Step? Are your food thoughts starting to diminish? Are you becoming more aware of their presence and ignoring rather than indulging them? How are you coming with busting your food romanticism? Are you starting to think more pragmatically about food? Are you telling yourself the truth about what food can and can't give you? Has this realization helped you to recognize when the Child is on the scene and ignore her dictates? Are you practicing your kung fus for cravings and emotional eating?

What about the Second Step? Are you starting to eat healthier? If you have been eating a healthier diet, your taste buds should be adjusting to it nicely. Wholesome fruits, vegetables, grains, and protein should be tasting pretty darn spectacular by now. Are you allowing yourself some treat foods that (ideally) have some nutritional value to make things a little more interesting? If you're still eating some junk, that's okay, too. As the grown-up in your new relationship with food, you'll need to gauge your own junk quotient. This work is about *you* deciding how to feed your body for the rest of your life. It's not another diet that you're adding to your resume.

What about the Third Step? Are you bringing more awareness to your eating—just eating while you're eating? Weighing yourself regularly to track your progress? Eating slowly? Making friends with hunger? Eating reasonable portion sizes?

What about the Fourth Step? Have you been able to question the stressful thoughts that ravage your self-esteem, speak your truth from the place of the Wise Witness, and be kind and gentle with yourself when you've spoken the ego's truth instead? Are you having more fun, doing things you enjoy and are good at, and taking time to rest and feed your soul?

Remember, you don't need to do everything all at once. This is your process and you decide when to implement changes. You're embarking on a new way of living, creating new habits, so it's perfectly okay to take it slow.

Some of the steps will be easier for you than others, and there may be some components you don't need to implement at all in order to feel healed and relegate weight problems to a distant memory. For example, my relationship with food is healed and is now very pragmatic, but sometimes I still nibble while I'm cooking. It's okay because I don't suffer over it and my weight and health aren't impacted. Other people may need to fully commit to a non-nibbling stance.

I had to be steadfast about the First and Second Steps, Wise Thinking and Wise Food Choices. I frankly don't believe that anyone can be nonchalant about problematic food thinking. Nip those romantic food thoughts in the bud! Indulging in excessive food thinking creates desire and leads to overeating and eating the wrong foods. I could not have taken a namby-pamby stance about sugar and chocolate and healed my compulsion to eat those foods.

If you're not addicted to any particular foods, this may not be true for you. You may be able to keep more junk food in your life because you can limit your consumption and keep it under control. *Skinny*

Thinking tells you the truth about food and your thinking, but how you use it is up to you. You become a grown-up and level with yourself about what you're willing to do. But remember, the Five Steps are about freedom, not about becoming perfect, so be gentle with yourself.

Hopefully, you're well on your way to taking your life back from nagging thoughts about food and weight, and are ready to learn about the Fifth Step, Wise Relationship with Your Body. Creating a wise relationship with your body means accepting your body just as it is and allowing change to happen from a place of tenderness rather than forcing your body to change as a result of the Critic's loathing or the Dreamer's fantasizing. It may seem contradictory for me to suggest that you accept your body and at the same time decide to lose weight to improve your health. But to reject the reality of your current body size is to suffer, and it doesn't even help you lose weight! Both accepting your current size and changing your diet to achieve a healthier body are expressions of honoring and loving yourself.

This is where the *Skinny Thinking* approach differs from diets that actually reinforce the voices of the Critic and the Dreamer. The key is noticing where the impulse to change comes from. If it's a loving impulse, it's coming from the heart and supports a new, wiser relationship with the body and leads to healing. If it's an egoic impulse, it leads to suffering.

Can you even imagine what it would feel like to accept your body right now? It's a radical idea that doesn't even occur to most women. But not only is it possible, it's the likely outcome of creating these new habits. So why not start right now? Close your eyes, take a deep breath, set the intention, and ask for help to be able to accept your body exactly as it is now, in this moment.

The Birth of a Core Belief about the Body

Negative beliefs about our bodies often develop early in childhood. They're reinforced throughout our teen years and, by the time we're out of high school, many of us have become card-carrying members of the culture of body loathing. As you read my story, think back to the events that formed your own core beliefs about your body.

What Price Beauty?

Growing up, my neighborhood friend Stephanie always managed to have a tan, even in Park Forest, Illinois. The boys took notice, tripping over each other to tag her, tease her, and sneak up behind her to pull her pretty brown hair. My hair was a mess of wiry springs, Stephanie's a silky train that dazzled onlookers when she ran.

When I compared our two bodies, I noticed that mine was shorter, thicker, and paler than hers, and quickly came to the conclusion that my body was too fat. Although I couldn't do anything about the wiry springs or being short, I decided I could rectify the thicker and paler (in the summertime, at least).

I asked Effie, our housekeeper, if she knew about diets, and she swore that the lemon juice diet would melt away my unwanted pounds. All I had to do was drink lemon juice before every meal. Effie made me a glass. I took a sip of the sour stuff, promptly decided that the lemon juice diet was yucky, and gave up!

A few months later, my mother took me shopping for pants one day. As I was trying on a pair, I heard the saleslady whisper to my mother, "She's got quite a hip on her. She's definitely going to need the next size up." I was 10 and this was the first time that I'd heard a remark like that directed at my body. My hips were too big, and they were the wrong size for my body. Pants weren't made for bodies like mine, I decided. If my waist fit into one size, the hips were too tight. In the next size up, the hips fit well, but I could stick my whole fist inside the waistband!

At school a few years later, my friends and I began judging our bodies in the locker room, sharing negative thoughts like "My hair is too thin"; "My thighs are too fat"; and "I hate my freckles." Together, we invented our own language of body loathing and honed it throughout our teens. The unwritten rule was: Say only negative things about your own body and disagree when others make negative comments about theirs.

This was also about the time when it became cool to go on a diet. One day during lunch, I decided to buy an ice cream sandwich and asked if anyone else at my table wanted one. My friends looked at each other in disbelief, as if I'd asked if they wanted twice the homework. I quickly learned that they were watching their weight and that dessert was out of the question.

As I entered into this rite of passage called dieting, I became a member of a new society, one preoccupied with comparison. We compared notes on diet rituals and cheered each other on as we tried to achieve perfect bodies—that is, of course, until one of the girls succeeded and the rest of us looked inferior by comparison. Once we started dieting, my girlfriends and I were no longer just friends, we were rivals in the "who has the cutest clothes, best figure, and hottest boyfriend" competition.

As we transitioned from girlhood to womanhood, our bodies became the ultimate way we measured our self-worth. Because we couldn't hide them, there was no denying how we were faring in our struggle to achieve a thin body. The prettiest girls with the best bodies got attention from the boys, and the rest of us suffered the humiliating fate of invisibility.

A Writ of Body Attachment

In the criminal justice system, a warrant for someone's arrest is called a writ of body attachment. In spiritual parlance, body attachment is the belief that *you are the body*. In both examples, body attachment equates with a loss of freedom: physical freedom in the case of the criminal justice system and essential freedom—the freedom to experience our true nature—in the case of the spirit. According to Hindu philosophy, the notion "I am the body" lies at the root of all human suffering.

When we believe that we are our body, we think that when it gets old, we're old, when it's fat and out of shape, we're fat and out of shape. No one around us questions this belief and neither do we because it's easy to get caught up in the messages of our culture and forget the simple truth: we are spiritual beings having a human experience, not the other way around. Your body may be heavier than other bodies, but fat can never be *who you are*.

Here is how you became identified with your body: Starting with your name, you were taught to think of yourself as a person separate from others. Soon, you learned that you were either a girl or a boy person. As you got older, you noticed that when your particular body fell down and skinned its knee, you felt the pain, but your sister didn't. Over time, you moved from not being identified with your body (as when you were a baby) to complete body identification. This change was twofold:

1. First, you linked the notion of self with the body. You looked in the mirror and acknowledged, "This reflected image is me, not my brother, my mother, or my dog, but me."

2. Second, you innocently attributed certain meanings, some positive and some negative, to the body and its gender, appearance, size, shape, and function. For example: "My body is female, *and that means* the world will take me less seriously. My body has long fingers, *and that means* I'm well suited to playing the piano. My body has big, round eyes, *and that means* I'm pretty. I have a small chin, *and that means* I'm weak. I'm overweight, *and that means* no one will ever love me, and I will always be alone and unhappy."

In addition, you learned that bodies of your gender are supposed to look a certain way, and that yours either did or didn't. Eventually, there was a moment of reckoning when you stood before the mirror, took a good hard look, and decided how you measured up. If you decided you didn't measure up, in that moment, you created a negative body image.

Listening to the voices of the Dreamer and the Critic as you got older, you likely put tremendous pressure on yourself to be the best you could be. For women, this desire often extends to body size. You believed that people would either think well or ill of you, judge or envy you, or desire or reject you based on how your body looked. You were subjected to a daily barrage of media images of young, beautiful, thin women who seemed to be leading happy, glamorous lives, and this reinforced your belief. The implicit message you received was that to be successful, you had to look like them.

This pressure to conform to cultural standards of beauty and thinness doesn't feel good. When you have negative beliefs about your body because you're listening to the Critic, and you decide that because your body isn't up to par, then neither are you, you suffer.

"But hold on," you may say. "I don't really believe those things about my body." And you may be right, but what about your unconscious beliefs? If your goal is to create a healthy relationship with your body, then becoming conscious of those unconscious beliefs is important. Start by asking to be shown those beliefs. Then, be on the lookout for any insights that may surface. Once you identify the beliefs, you can take them to inquiry and weaken their negative influence.

To begin to detach from the idea that you are your body, revisit the idea of your body as a car, ferrying you from point A to point B. It's merely at your service, helping you get around and experience life in the material world. Your job is to keep it clean, fueled, and maintained. When you use a car to get from place to place, you don't confuse it with yourself. You don't think you *are* the car, right? So why would you think that you are your body?

You might think that because you experience your body's sensations. To challenge this idea, ask, "Who is seeing this body?" The answer is, of course, "I am." If you're the one seeing this body, how could it be you? Whenever you notice that you're identified with your body, take a moment to remember the truth—it's just your earth-exploring vehicle—and snap out of it.

Fear and Desire

The root of our desire to get pleasure from food is fear. If we inquire into the beliefs that underlie our stress, agitation, anger, and sadness, we discover the fear of loss. In my case, because I decided that my body was flawed, I was afraid that I would lose my chance to have a happy life. To distract myself from my fear, I desired pleasure, overate, and gained weight. My fear of loss translated into a fear of the negative consequences that I attributed to being overweight—humiliation, loneliness, and low self-esteem. Out of these fears grew my desire to get thin.

After reaching my goal weight through dieting, I couldn't rest because I was always afraid of gaining weight again. This fear created a desire for pleasure, and I was back on the merry-go-round again. This was the perfect setup for yo-yo dieting and endless weight gain and loss. Thankfully, I was eventually able to end this cycle by questioning my negative beliefs and learning to stop romanticizing food.

What Your Beliefs about Body Weight Mean about You

Forcing stressful, unconscious body beliefs out of the shadows and into the light of day allows you to see that they never tell the whole truth. This discovery is the first step in their dissolution. When they dissolve, there's nothing left to trigger painful emotions like anger, shame, fear, and sadness, and that can be a huge relief.

Negative emotions sap our energy and are the biggest triggers for eating for comfort and pleasure. The more you can allow your negative beliefs about food, your body, life, others, or yourself to dissolve, the fewer negative emotions you'll create, and the less you'll be moved to eat emotionally.

In the last chapter, we explored some of your beliefs about eating to satisfy emotional needs. Now, take a few minutes to explore your beliefs about your body and your weight. Circle any of the following beliefs that ring true for you so that you can question them later. My body:

- ❀ Is out of control.
- ❀ Is insatiable.
- ❀ Has to be governed with an iron fist.
- ❀ Is programmed to make me fat.
- ❀ Is fat and ugly.

What Carrying More Weight Means about Me

Next, look at the meaning you've given to your beliefs about carrying more body weight. Circle what is true for you.

What It Means about My Character

- ❀ I'm weak and have no willpower.
- ❀ I'm a hopeless failure.
- ❀ I'm not lovable.

What It Means to Others (Friends, Family, Colleagues)

- ❀ I'm lazy.
- ❀ I'm not living up to my potential.
- ❀ I'm someone to look down upon, who's not in their "league."
- ❀ I'm gluttonous.
- ❀ I'm a loser.
- ❀ I'm an example of how not to live.
- ❀ My body is:
  - ○ Dumpy.
  - ○ Asexual.
  - ○ Disgusting.
  - ○ A turnoff.

What It Means about How I Live My Life

- ❁ I'll stop shopping for clothes.
- ❁ I'll avoid mirrors.
- ❁ I'll stop socializing.
- ❁ I'll stop trying to find a partner.
- ❁ I'll avoid thinner friends and family because I don't want to be compared to them.

What It Means about My Ability to Be in Relationships

- ❁ I won't be able to attract the kind of partner I want.
- ❁ My partner will always be on the lookout for someone thinner.

What It Means about My Career

- ❁ I won't have the respect of my subordinates, peers, or superiors.
- ❁ People at work will assume I lack self-esteem and willpower.
- ❁ I'll lose out on promotions.
- ❁ I'll never live up to my potential.

What It Means to My Parents

- ❁ They will be ashamed of me.
- ❁ They will wonder where they went wrong with me.
- ❁ They will feel like failures.

What Carrying Less Weight Means about Me

In this section, you'll investigate negative beliefs about being thin. If you think you don't have any negative beliefs about being thin, think again. This section can be quite an eye-opener. Circle each of the following beliefs that ring true for you:

What It Means about My Character

- I'm weak and easily succumb to societal pressures.
- I'm not lovable.

What It Means to Others (Friends, Family, Colleagues)

- They envy me and hate me for being thin.
- They want to have sex with me, and I don't want that.
- They think I'm vain and self-involved.
- They think my body is:
  - Asexual.
  - Wiry.
  - Masculine.
  - Unappealing.
  - A turnoff.
  - Hard and angular.

What It Means to My Parents

- They worry about me.
- They wonder where they went wrong with me that I am so consumed with being thin.

What It Means about How I Live My Life

- I won't be able to hide anymore.
- I won't have any more excuses to avoid living my life.
- I won't be able to live in my future fantasy world anymore. I'll have to face my life as it is.
- I'll have to take risks, and I might fail.
- I'll have to give up food as my primary source of emotional nourishment.

- To stay thin, I'll have to starve myself and give up the foods I like.
- I won't be able to enjoy food.
- Staying at my natural weight will be a constant struggle, so I'll always be stressed out, hungry, and unhappy.
- Being at my natural weight equals deprivation.
- I'll love looking at myself in the mirror and become totally superficial and self-absorbed.
- I'll spend too much money on clothes and have to declare bankruptcy.
- I'll be unhappy because I'll live in fear of gaining the weight back.
- The people I love won't love me anymore.
- I'll feel like a failure.

What It Means about My Ability to Be in Relationships

- I'll feel exposed and vulnerable without my fat armor to protect me.
- I won't be able to attract the kind of partner I want.
- I'll get too much sexual attention and won't know how to fend it off.
- I won't be loved.
- I'll end up alone.
- I'll stop trying to find a partner.
- I'll avoid heavier friends and family members because I won't want to be compared to them. I'll worry that they'll feel jealous and uncomfortable being around me.

What It Means about My Career

- I won't have the respect of my colleagues.
- I'll lose out on promotions because people will see me as a sex object and not take me seriously.
- I'll never live up to my potential.

Inquiry for Negative Beliefs about the Body

Now that you've identified many of your body judgments and seen how they've affected your life, here's your chance to loosen their grip on you. Look at these examples of negative body beliefs to see how inquiry can weaken them.

Negative Belief: I can't be happy unless I'm thin.

Inquiry:

1. **Can I know beyond a shadow of a doubt that this is true?** Close your eyes. Let the question sink in so that the answer can arise from within you rather than rushing to come up with the answer. The ego tends to jump in with what it thinks is true. If your answer is yes, you can absolutely know that you can only be happy if your body is thin, ask yourself if you can predict the future. Can you really know how you would feel? Even if the answer is "Yes, I know I can only be happy if I'm thin," move on to the next phase of inquiry.

2. **What is the opposite of this belief?** I can be happy if I'm not thin. **Could this new belief be as true or truer?** This is at least as true. **What is your evidence for this?** I was thin a few years ago. I liked how my body looked, but I was obsessed with not gaining weight again. I couldn't enjoy myself because I was always worried and stressed out.

Negative Belief: I hate my body.

Inquiry:

1. **Can I know beyond a shadow of a doubt that this is true?**
2. **What is the opposite of this belief?** I love my body. **Could this new belief be as true or truer? What is your evidence for this?** I love my body because:
   - It keeps me alive and functioning in the world.

- It allows me to move from place to place.
- Its skin lets me experience a cool breeze on a hot day.
- It has good vision and hearing.
- Its teeth are strong and healthy.

If you thought you hated your body, could you find evidence to support the opposite belief: I love my body? If you were able to see how you actually do appreciate your body, what happened? Was there any softening of your original negative belief? If so, you've begun to heal your conditioning about your body. It's like a row of dominoes: once you tip over that first negative belief, it won't be long before the whole line goes!

At your own pace, go back and take each of the negative beliefs you circled in the last two sections to inquiry. Set a goal of questioning one belief each day, and see what happens to your relationship with your body.

Pursuing the Perfect Body: The Road to Hell

I used to believe I couldn't be happy if I wasn't at my ideal weight. Caught up in the world of the Dreamer, I believed that if I were thin, all my problems would melt away. Dreaming about a future like that can be fun, but it's insidious because it means that if your body doesn't look the way you think it should—even if you have all the trappings of a successful life—you're guaranteed to suffer.

If you've reached your ideal weight at some point in your life, did it make you happy? You attracted more attention and admiration, but did that translate into happiness? Did you worry about maintaining your weight? Were the partners you attracted the kind of people you wanted to be with?

Over the last 35 years, my body has been 10 to 30 pounds heavier than my ego preferred, so I suffered. I struggled, strived, lost weight, and was happy for brief intervals. Of course, the ego attributed this happiness to my new, thinner body. But the real reason I was happy was that, in those intervals, I got a break from striving! My desire for a thinner body caused me to suffer, and when I reached my goal weight, the striving ceased for a bit, and so did my suffering.

When I was heavy, I didn't understand that *the thought* that my body didn't look right was causing my pain, not my body's appearance. Without the thought, the body was just doing what it did—breathing, walking, sleeping, and there was no suffering. What was having a problem with my body's so-called imperfect size? None other than the ego, of course!

I wasn't able to see that I'd had the perfect body all along! I have always had the perfect body through which to learn and experience life. You don't have to wait to be happy until your ego blesses your image in the mirror. You can be happy right now. You know this is true because you've experienced moments of happiness, regardless of your body size. *You're happy when you experience life directly, without analyzing or judging it;* and you suffer when you believe thoughts that say you look bad.

The desire to be thin, when it comes from wanting to be admired, causes suffering and creates an "us versus them" worldview. In wanting to be above the crowd, we isolate ourselves from other people and move away from love. The truth is: Most other people don't really care how you look; they're too busy worrying about how *they* look. The only one keeping score is your pesky ego!

Thankfully, we can step out of the Critic and the Dreamer and relate to our body from the Wise Witness. When we do that, it's easy to follow intuitions that move us toward health, moderation, and balance. The Wise Witness accepts our body being overweight and, at the same time, intends that we bring our body back to a healthy weight.

The idea that a perfect body will make you happy is just a thought, a belief. If you've reached your ideal weight at some point in your life, did it make you happy? Perhaps you attracted more attention and admiration, but did that translate into happiness? Did you worry about maintaining your weight? Were the partners you attracted the kind of people you wanted to be with?

The key to becoming free from this belief is to see it for what it is—a lie, or at best a partial truth. You do this by remembering the times you've been happy at a heavier weight and unhappy at a lighter weight. Then, you can begin to dis-identify with the body altogether, whatever its weight. That's true freedom.

Stressed and Obsessed

The myth of thinness is: If we achieve the body of our dreams, we'll live happily ever after. After all, models and movie stars seem to lead charmed lives. So it's natural to assume that if our bodies looked like theirs, our lives would be great, too.

The rub is that media images of hyperthin female bodies create an impossible standard for most women to attain. For diet programs, gyms, and spas, this myth means money in the till. It keeps us striving, and if we're striving, we're also buying. But after the diet ends or the gym membership runs out, the Child resurfaces, tempting us with the pleasure food we've been missing and, of course, we regain the weight.

As a society, we're body obsessed. Unwittingly, we contribute to this obsession through our own behavior. To avoid that, the next time you see a friend, try to refrain from commenting on her appearance or weight and comment on her inner state instead.

Oprah Winfrey, one of the truly iconic figures of our time, admitted that no matter how much success, fame, or money she had, none of it mattered if she couldn't fit into her clothes. If she couldn't control her eating, she couldn't be happy. Her Critic told her that if she couldn't manage her weight, she was a failure.

Our Critic tells us the same thing. Of course, it has a vested interest in keeping us feeling bad about ourselves because if we're suffering, we're more likely to follow its plans. The ego loves its own cycle—striving, followed by success, followed by failure, followed by more striving, on and on until we die, having never reached our happily ever after.

Is It Worth the Suffering?

If you accept being overweight right now, what does that mean? Does it mean you'll slide into being fatter and fatter and never be thin again? Can you try to accept that your body weighs what it weighs right now? That doesn't mean that it won't ever weigh less, and it certainly doesn't mean that it will weigh this much for the rest of your life!

If you're suffering over not having the perfect body, over not achieving the Dreamer's dream, ask yourself, "Is it worth the suffering? Does it really matter?" What would happen if you just let yourself be the way you are—just for now?

What does your excess weight mean to you? It's important to look at what the extra weight means because *the meaning you're giving it is causing your suffering.* Who is the one who cares that you might not look as attractive carrying the extra weight, the ego or your true self? It's the ego, of course.

Can you accept the ego's preference? Can you accept not liking your excess weight? Is it worth the suffering that resisting the way your body looks right now causes you? Really look at this because *suffering doesn't change anything.* Not liking your body doesn't change anything. It only causes you pain. For this reason, resistance is an irrational stance. If your body is this way, you might as well like it. Why spend even one second evaluating it? It doesn't serve you.

Trying to lose weight for health reasons, to look and feel better is one thing, but trying to create a perfect body is quite another. If you want a perfect body, it's important to ask yourself, "Is that where I want to put my energy? Is that what I want to focus on?" Striving for the perfect body takes a tremendous amount of time, energy, and money. Look at what celebrities go through to look the way they do. If that's what's important to you, go for it, but realize that there's a cost.

That cost is all the attention you end up giving to your looks. Your life becomes all about appearances. You only have so much time and energy, so it's important to ask yourself, "Does looking perfect matter? How much does it matter?"

Looking perfect matters an awful lot to the ego because it wants to be admired for being beautiful, disciplined, and special. But there's no happiness in it because being admired for physical beauty comes paired with the suffering of trying to hold on to it. Aging robs even the most exquisitely beautiful people of their looks.

It can be hard to love people who look so perfect. In fact, they sometimes lack the poise, calm, and inner beauty that others who are less beautiful possess because they've focused so much on outer beauty. Inner beauty and alignment with your true self are what make people want to be close to you.

Think of all the people you know who aren't beautiful but are totally lovable. Isn't it true that you love them all the more for their imperfections? *Being at peace with how you look rather than obsessing over it* is actually much more attractive than outer beauty.

It's one thing to care about the health of your body, but there's no fulfillment or happiness in caring so much about your appearance. Try putting your attention and energy into serving others, being present with them, loving and accepting them, and seeing their inner beauty. Once you do this, you'll forget about striving to achieve the perfect body and stop suffering because you haven't. You have only so much energy and so much time. Where will you put your attention—on the inner or the outer? The outer is a dead end.

A New Relationship with the Mirror

Most of us look in the mirror through the eyes of the Critic. As we look, we zero in on our problem areas: "Am I getting old? How do my thighs look? Is that a new wrinkle? Is my jawline sagging?" The Critic sees flaws and, because all bodies are flawed in some way, mirrors are its perfect tool.

Once the Critic identifies your flaws, it urges you to imagine how others will see you. Then it comes up with a plan to fix you, fueled by the Dreamer's fantasies about being admired and the wonderful life you could have if you looked the way it tells you you should. If you're suffering over what you see in the mirror, in that moment, you're identifying with the ego.

From the Wise Witness, we can forge a new relationship with the mirror by simply not looking too closely. That means doing what we need to do, like brushing our teeth or hair, and then moving on. It means looking in the mirror briefly and not scrutinizing, evaluating, judging, or imagining what other people are seeing.

If you can step back and become aware of *that which is looking*, you align with the Wise Witness and connect with its compassion for the contracted part of you that's unhappy with what it's seeing. Once you become aware of your negative relationship with the image in the mirror and the suffering created by the harsh, rejecting, perhaps even violent way you've been scrutinizing it, you can choose to stop any negative self-talk and develop a kinder relationship with the image. Negative thoughts such as "I don't like it"; "I want to change it"; and "That's awful!" aren't us, they're our conditioning. The more we realize that the mirror brings out the Critic, the more we can work to develop a different relationship with the image by being very gentle with it.

The Wise Witness knows that this two-dimensional representation of the body isn't you. Only when you look deeply into the eyes of the reflection do you get a taste of what you really are—radiant spaciousness, beyond name and form.

When we're away from mirrors, it's easier to become more aligned with *what is looking out from our eyes* (our true self) than with *what our eyes see*. When we align with the Wise Witness, we experience ourselves looking rather than as objects being looked at. When we believe we're objects, it allows the Critic to rush in and judge us. If you want to stop suffering over how your body looks, avoiding long looks in the mirror can really help.

The lesson we can learn from body-weight issues and aging is that our inner beauty—our authenticity and comfort in our own skin—is what makes us beautiful. To catch a glimpse of your inner beauty, that which is looking out from your eyes, try this exercise:

> *Look into your eyes in the mirror for 15 to 20 minutes and see what happens!*

Through this exercise, it's possible to experience the truth of what you are because your visage gets lost in your looking. When you look into your eyes for a long time, it helps you break through the illusion of identifying yourself with your body. Is that face yours? Is it real? If so, why does it keep changing? You think your face looks a certain way but as you keep looking, you may see it morph into many other faces. The truth is that you're all of those faces—the beautiful and not so beautiful—and none of them.

This exercise helps you see that you aren't just one image. After all, no one image of you has stayed the same throughout your life. What you're looking at just comes and goes—the beautiful and the ugly all appear. What's *looking* is what's true and real. The image, the appearance, is transitory. When we're at peace with that, other people relax and become very comfortable with us. We transmit ease and contentment when we're at peace with ourselves and how we look, and that allows others to be at peace, too.

The Goldilocks Approach

The perfect body is the one that's appearing in this moment, the one that's reflected back in the mirror. To stop suffering over how your body looks, I recommend the Goldilocks approach: "This body is not too thin or too fat but juuust right for this moment." Can you let your body be the way that it is right now?

The truth is, your body is the way it is in this moment. You can't change that fact. Whoops! It's too late anyway; the moment is already over. To reject this reality is to suffer. You can either be at this weight and accept it or be at this weight and suffer. Which will you choose: freedom and happiness or suffering? It's up to you. If you can accept your body for now, it leaves you free to move forward from a rational place of health and balance. Acceptance of your body in the moment does not mean your body will never change. But if you resist your body in the moment, if you hate it, you'll stay stuck for sure.

"But wait," you may say. "How can I accept what I don't like? If I don't like this body, is it still possible to accept it?" Yes. You simply accept that your body is how it is right now. It may not be your preference, but if you can allow it, you will move out of resistance. If you can let it be okay that the ego doesn't like how your body looks right now, you are outside of the ego. You are noticing the resistance and accepting it. It may seem subtle, but there's a Gulf of Mexico between thinking *you are* the flawed body and noticing that the ego doesn't like how your body looks.

Replacing Negative Thoughts with Positive Ones

The culture of body loathing is pervasive among women, and if we don't partake, we're suspect. Yet the price of participation is steep: reinforcing and perpetuating negative body images and cultural messages. This often leaves us and our sisters miserable.

To help heal your negative body-image issues, try this exercise: Simply replace any negative body thoughts with their opposites. For example, if your thought is "I hate my stomach," replace it with "I love my stomach." If your thought is "My skin is too wrinkled," replace it with "I love the lines on this face." Even if you don't believe these positive thoughts at first, just keep repeating them and finding supporting examples. For instance, "I love this stomach that stretched to accommodate my pregnancies" contains a compelling reason for loving your stomach and creates a positive new story that replaces your negative one. Set an intention to replace negative thoughts with positive ones. The more you do that, the less negative thoughts will be able to suck you in, and pretty soon, they won't be able to enter your airspace undetected at all!

As you separate your sense of self from your image of the body, you're more able to view the body as just your earth-exploring vehicle, not a statement of your worth. You don't have to take its weight personally. As you begin to dis-identify with your body, the body that appears in the mirror will seem to be no more yours than the mail carrier's. You call it yours, but perhaps it's only out on loan—so why not care for it as you might a favorite car and stop identifying with it?

"What if I stop seeing my body as who I am? Then what? Who will I be then?" you may ask. Great question! Are you willing to find out? What do you have to lose? You may discover that the only thing you ever had to lose was your suffering!

The Miracle of Acceptance

While I was attending The School for The Work with Byron Katie, Katie engaged a woman who had said she believed that she was too fat. In their dialogue, Katie remarked on the absurdity of the woman wanting her body to be different than it was in that moment. As I contemplated Katie's words, I felt something shift inside me. I had never really appreciated the clarity of this simple notion before. Wishing that my body were different than it was right then was ludicrous—completely and utterly insane! I could wish all I wanted, but in that moment, *the condition of my body was undeniably and irrevocably what it was. It couldn't be an ounce lighter or heavier nor a millimeter larger or smaller. My skin couldn't be a shade darker or lighter nor smoother or more wrinkled. The age of my body couldn't be a second older or younger. It all made sense. In a millisecond, something inside me recognized this truth so profoundly that all identification with my body vanished.*

In the blink of an eye, this powerful locus of identity—my body—no longer made any sense to me. It was an object, no different than my chair or the plants in the room. It bore no relationship to me other than its role as trusty servant, squiring me around and allowing me to experience the world through its five senses.

"This is the healing power of the moment," I thought to myself. "The only thing that is ever asked of us in this journey of self-discovery is to be present in this moment. Without warning or fanfare, grace descends and miracles happen." In a single moment, this body, formerly a source of misery, was fully and completely accepted. I can't even say that I did it. It just happened.

To test this stunning change in perspective, I went up to my room and undressed. Until then, seeing my reflection had been so painful that I had steered clear of mirrors and bathed only in dim light, but there I was, looking at it in broad daylight! My eyes lovingly glided over the form, giving special attention to the places that had once been sources of aversion: the spongy fat underneath the skin in the belly, the ripples and bumps of the cellulite on the thighs, the age spots on the legs and arms, and the wrinkles on the face. Amazingly, I had only tender feelings for this faithful servant. It was as if I were seeing it for the first time. I realized that by perceiving this body through my negative judgments about it, I'd missed it entirely.

Detaching from the belief that "I am the body" created some interesting hypotheticals for me. First, I thought about a potent old fear—being naked in public. I'd had so many nightmares about this, but now, it held no power over me. I could have stripped down in front of the entire school of 320 people if I'd had to, and it wouldn't have phased me a bit!

Silly as it may sound, one of the first thoughts I had after dis-identifying with the body was, "Wow, this is great! I won't ever have to hold my stomach in again!" All of my self-consciousness about how my body looked in clothes or what anyone thought about it had vanished. None of that interested me anymore. Paying attention to clothes or how my body looked seemed about as exciting as ruminating about what kind of packaging breakfast cereal came in. This body had nothing to do with me. My role was to be grateful for its service and to care for it like I cared for our car.

Next, I noticed that I wasn't judging other people's bodies either. This was very strange because my mind had formerly been full of those kinds of

*thoughts. If I wasn't judging my own body, I was judging someone else's.
Now, I couldn't find a body that was "too" anything. Ideas like "She's too
heavy"; "She's too short"; and "Her head is out of proportion to her body"
just didn't arise. All I could see was beauty and perfection. It was like I had
gone to sleep one night and woken up inside someone else's head!*

Exercise: Seeing the Body in This Moment

*Find a quiet place to be alone, close your eyes, take a few deep
breaths, and relax. Feel the flesh of your body and sense its shape.
Ask yourself the following: "Is it possible for my body to be any
different than it is right now—in this moment?" Really let the
question sink in. Simply be present with it. Feel the absurdity of
wishing or expecting your body to be different. Next, ask yourself,
"Is it okay for my body to be the way it is right now?"*

After my discovery, I queried a teacher of mine about how this
miracle of dis-identification could have happened. He reminded me
that I'd been praying to be free of body-related suffering for a long time.
For years, I'd been attending body-image workshops, performing self-
inquiry, and just plain praying and asking for help with this issue. He
suggested that perhaps all of my work and praying had finally brought
the healing that I'd hoped for.

Becoming free from body identification is like chopping down
a tree. We swing the axe over and over again, chipping away at the
seemingly impenetrable trunk. From all outer appearances, our efforts
have little impact, but we keep swinging. Then, swinging the axe for
the thousandth time, without warning, one unremarkable blow fells
the mighty tree. In the same way, this apparently intractable issue can
topple in a moment.

Back at home, still dis-identified with my body, I hoped that my
body-image suffering was over. But although my relationship with my
body had changed, my relationship with food hadn't. As a result, I

gained weight, and my ego immediately started saying a lot of unpleasant things to me. As I listened to the Critic's derisive thoughts rather than questioning them, I began to believe them. I started to suffer again and my body identification returned. Thankfully, many years and inquiry sessions later, my body identification has gradually diminished again. Though it has not completely vanished, I rarely suffer over my body's appearance these days.

Looking at the Body Objectively

Your body simply is the way it is in this moment. That's reality. Wishing and hoping for it to be different is a losing and painful proposition. It might break a limb in the next 30 seconds or go on a diet tomorrow and become smaller, but why suffer by resisting the truth of this moment?

Look at your body objectively. Pretend that it belongs to someone else and evaluate it factually, using neutral descriptors. Here are some examples of neutral body descriptions:

- This body is five feet, three inches tall.
- The hair is long, blond, and wavy.
- The skin is pale.
- The legs are muscular.
- The shoulders are broad.
- The fingers are long.

See if you can come up with a similar description for your body. Imagine you are a scientist describing a body in a professional report. This exercise can help you experience what it would be like to view your body without judgment or identification.

Honoring Yourself

Close your eyes and find the part of you that's struggled with eating, weight, and body-image issues for so long. See the suffering you've endured. Remember the times you've experienced self-loathing, castigation, and shame for being caught in the crossfire between the desire for pleasure food and the desire to be thin. Feel compassion for your suffering and honor your perseverance in looking for a way out. Honor the humility that has allowed you to open yourself to a new perspective, one that runs counter to conventional wisdom. See how you've tried to create moderation and balance in your life, struggled to overcome weight and body-image issues, worked on yourself, tried different diets, read self-help books, and endured the negative comments of others and the Critic. Take a moment to honor yourself and feel grateful for your fortitude and perseverance while grappling with some of life's most difficult issues. Congratulate yourself for having the courage to move beyond your old patterns and try something new.

Skinny Thinking is not a magic pill. Appreciate yourself for having the patience to endure a process that has its own timing and *is not instantaneous*. In our culture, we've come to expect immediate results, but compulsive patterns that have been reinforced over many years aren't likely to vanish overnight. Please continue to be patient and tolerant with yourself. It takes time to incorporate these new perspectives and habits.

Now that you've come this far, you're at the point of no return. If you've already been putting these new concepts into practice, you're probably beginning to taste the freedom awaiting you. But even if you aren't ready to put any of the steps into practice, just reading about this perspective has irrevocably altered your thinking. By learning this new perspective and practicing the Five Steps, you're moving toward a healthy, balanced relationship with food.

Read this book over and over again so that the ideas presented become second nature. Let them become your new way of thinking about eating, weight, and yourself. The key to healing your body-image issues is changing the way you think about your body. If you can change the way you think about it, what it represents to you, and how you relate to the image in the mirror, you will experience freedom and happiness.

Once you've seen the truth, you can never go back to believing the lie. You can never go back to seeing food, your body, and your relationship with them in the same way. Congratulations! It's only a matter of time before your food, weight, and body-image issues are distant memories.

Surrender

At the beginning of this book, I told you that it is possible to live without measuring your self-worth by the vicissitudes of the bathroom scale. That it is possible to leave body and food-related suffering behind for good. My confidence in those statements is based on my healing of a deeply entrenched, dysfunctional relationship with eating and my body.

Surrender is an alien concept in Western culture. If we want something—anything—we're taught to go out and get it because that's what winners do. Our dreams are limited only by our imaginations. Once we settle on a goal, we follow it unwaveringly to completion. Heroes in the movies never give up, and neither do we.

Growing up, we learn expressions like "When the going gets tough, the tough get going" and "If it were easy, everyone would do it." Losers surrender. Winners never quit. They tough it out until their last breath.

Surrender is more of an acknowledgement than an action. It happens when we stop our habitual behavior, take stock of things, and realize that forcing, pushing, and controlling our way through life has never brought happiness and satisfaction. It's stepping back and looking at ourselves with tenderness and compassion, the way we would look at a young child who accidentally broke a dish. Surrender is a gentle acknowledgement of how we innocently caused our own misery, and by virtue of that acknowledgement, an ending of our misery forever.

Contrary to the predominant cultural messages, surrender is an act of maturity, courage, compassion, self-love, and acceptance that says, "I accept this moment exactly as it is." When we see the whole truth about food and our bodies relative to our misunderstandings and false projections, that's surrender. When we earnestly set the intention and ask for help in healing our relationship with food and our bodies, that's surrender. Surrender is an act of humility, an acknowledgement that how we've been seeing things and behaving hasn't been working and has been causing us to suffer.

This acknowledgement is a major rite of passage. It allows us to move away from the Child, the Critic, and the Dreamer, and aligns us with our own inner wisdom, our Wise Witness. In this moment of clarity and recognition, miracles happen, and freedom is ours.

One day, without ceremony or fanfare, you'll realize that you can't remember the last time you had a worry about eating or your weight, that you can't remember the last time you paid attention to or suffered over a critical thought about your body, that these issues you thought you would take to your grave are finally healed. That is my prayer for you.

Wise Relationship with Your Body Check-in

Congratulations! You made it through all Five Steps! Appreciate yourself for your commitment to your own growth and healing. It takes tremendous courage to even think about changing your relationship to food, particularly if it's been your main source of comfort and pleasure. If you are putting some or all of the steps into practice, that's terrific! However, please don't be discouraged if you're not ready to start. An important part of this new relationship is learning to be gentle and kind to yourself. If this is the only message you take to heart and put into practice, it's a wonderful achievement.

Don't worry or chastise yourself if your diet isn't healthy yet or if you haven't been able to control your nibbling or ignore the voice of the Child, Dreamer, or Critic. You've created an emotional connection with food that takes time to reverse. Don't get discouraged if these steps take months or even years to complete. Be patient with yourself and remember, you don't need to be perfect. The rewards of following the

Five Steps will more than compensate for your efforts. Creating a new way of eating, relating to your body, and living will bring you freedom, peace of mind, and a healthier, slimmer body.

Chapter Summary

- ❑ The root of desire, which comes from the ego, is fear.
- ❑ When we inquire into the beliefs that underlie stress, agitation, anger, and sadness, we discover a fear of loss.
- ❑ Realizing that the beliefs we've been using to torture ourselves don't tell the whole truth undermines them.
- ❑ If we stop believing something, it has no power over us.
- ❑ The more painful the belief, the less truth it contains.
- ❑ If a thought makes you feel bad, then it's not true.
- ❑ You've always had the perfect body through which to learn and experience life.
- ❑ You don't have to wait to be happy until you have a so-called perfect body.
- ❑ Attaining the perfect, culturally sanctioned body doesn't lead to true happiness and may bring other undesirable consequences such as unwanted sexual attention, objectification, and worry about gaining weight again.
- ❑ Your true self accepts being overweight and, at the same time, intends that the body be brought back to a healthy weight.
- ❑ The ego pushes us to create a body that will attract attention and admiration.
- ❑ Disliking the way your body looks in this moment doesn't change anything. It's an irrational stance.
- ❑ There is no fulfillment or happiness in caring so much about how you look.
- ❑ Being at peace with how you look rather than obsessing over it is much more attractive to others.
- ❑ Mirrors reinforce identification with the body.

❑ The Wise Witness uses the mirror pragmatically, to help you do what you need to do before moving on.

❑ The Wise Witness knows that the image isn't who you are.

❑ When you're away from mirrors, you become more aligned with what's looking out from your eyes.

❑ Thoughts about the image in the mirror, such as "I don't like it" or "I want to change it," aren't us; they're our conditioning.

❑ When you focus on what is looking, you align with your true self and its compassion for the contracted part of you that's unhappy with what it's seeing.

❑ Your body and the image of it in the mirror are no more who you are than a tree is.

❑ The truth is that it doesn't matter what you look like.

❑ Inner beauty makes you beautiful.

❑ The Critic manifests as judgment, fear, and anxiety.

❑ Your true self generates intuitions that move you toward health, moderation, and balance.

❑ Changing negative patterns can take a long time because they have been reinforced over your entire life!

To-Do List

Check off any tasks that you have fully or partially completed:

❑ I've made a point of not looking too closely in the mirror.

❑ When I have looked in the mirror, I've avoided scrutinizing, evaluating, and judging, as well as imagining what other people are seeing.

❑ I've been working on breaking the habit of negative self-talk about my body and have been replacing any negative thoughts with positive thoughts.

❑ I did the mirror exercise.

❑ I asked for help to accept this body as it is, in this moment.

❑ I've been gentle and patient with myself.

RESOURCES

⊛ For information about *Skinny Thinking* Workshops, conference calls, and podcasts, and to receive the free e-newsletter, go to www.SkinnyThinking.com. Also, please follow me on Twitter and check out the Facebook fan group SKINNY THINKING! by Laura Katleman-Prue (www.facebook.com).

⊛ National Institute of Whole Health (NIWH), established in 1977, is the pioneer of Whole Health Education®, a Harvard hospital–tested model of health education and behavioral engagement. This outstanding integrative training is provided through a unique e-learning video format. The curriculum includes **evidence-based courses presented by nationally recognized health, nutrition, and medical experts,** filmed at renowned Boston-area hospitals and medical schools. These courses integrate medical science with natural health care and holistic concepts. For more information, contact NIWH at 888-354-HEAL (4325) or at info@wholehealtheducation.org.

RECOMMENDED READING

Robert Adams *Silence of the Heart*

Adyashanti *The Impact of Awakening: Excerpts from the Teachings of Adyashanti*

Byron Katie with Stephen Mitchell *A Thousand Names for Joy: Living in Harmony with the Way Things Are*

Loving What Is: Four Questions that Can Change Your Life

Gina Lake *Anatomy of Desire: How to Be Happy Even When You Don't Get What You Want*

Embracing the Now: Finding Peace and Happiness in What Is

Getting Free: How to Move Beyond Conditioning and Be Happy

Living in the Now: Reflections from Another Dimension About Being Happy in This One

Loving in the Moment

Radical Happiness: A Guide to Awakening

Return to Essence: How to Be in the Flow and Fulfill Your Life's Purpose

What About Now?: Reminders for Being in the Moment

Diana Schwarzbein and Nancy Deville *The Schwarzbein Principe: The Truth About Losing Weight, Being Healthy, and Feeling Younger*

Stuart Schwartz *The Great Undoing*

Dr. Bernie S. Siegel *365 Prescriptions for the Soul: Daily Messages of Inspiration, Hope, and Love*

Eckhart Tolle *The Power of Now: A Guide to Spiritual Enlightenment*

BUY A SHARE OF THE FUTURE IN YOUR COMMUNITY

These certificates make great holiday, graduation and birthday gifts that can be personalized with the recipient's name. The cost of one S.H.A.R.E. or one square foot is $54.17. The personalized certificate is suitable for framing and will state the number of shares purchased and the amount of each share, as well as the recipient's name. The home that you participate in "building" will last for many years and will continue to grow in value.

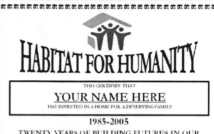

Here is a sample SHARE certificate:

YES, I WOULD LIKE TO HELP!

I support the work that Habitat for Humanity does and I want to be part of the excitement! As a donor, I will receive periodic updates on your construction activities but, more importantly, I know my gift will help a family in our community realize the dream of homeownership. **I would like to SHARE in your efforts against substandard housing in my community!** *(Please print below)*

PLEASE SEND ME _____ SHARES at $54.17 EACH = $ $_____

In Honor Of: _____

Occasion: (Circle One) HOLIDAY BIRTHDAY ANNIVERSARY

       OTHER: _____

Address of Recipient: _____

Gift From: _____ *Donor Address:* _____

Donor Email: _____

I AM ENCLOSING A CHECK FOR $ $_____ PAYABLE TO HABITAT FOR HUMANITY OR PLEASE CHARGE MY VISA OR MASTERCARD *(CIRCLE ONE)*

Card Number _____ Expiration Date: _____

Name as it appears on Credit Card _____ Charge Amount $ _____

Signature _____

Billing Address _____

Telephone # Day _____ Eve _____

PLEASE NOTE: Your contribution is tax-deductible to the fullest extent allowed by law.
Habitat for Humanity • P.O. Box 1443 • Newport News, VA 23601 • 757-596-5553
www.HelpHabitatforHumanity.org

LaVergne, TN USA
10 June 2010

185674LV00002B/2/P